Campbell's
Physiology Notes
for Nurses

Campbell's
Physiology Notes
for Nurses

John Campbell RGN, RMN, MSc
St Martin's College, Carlisle

WHURR PUBLISHERS
London & Philadelphia

© 2003 Whurr Publishers Ltd

First published 2003 by
Whurr Publishers Ltd
19b Compton Terrace, London N1 2UN, England
325 Chestnut Street, Philadelphia PA 19106, USA

Reprinted 2003, 2004, 2005 and 2006

British Library Cataloguing in Publication Data

A catalogue record for this book is available from the
British Library.

ISBN 1 86156 345 0

Printed and bound in the UK by Athenaeum Press Limited,
Gateshead, Tyne & Wear.

Contents

Preface

Welcome to these physiology notes. My name is John Campbell and I have been teaching nursing students for the past 12 years. Before entering nurse education I gained experience in several fields of nursing including psychiatry, theatres, neuromedicine, tropical medicine and intensive therapy units (ITUs). I still carry out clinical work in the ITU and accident and emergency (A and E) departments.

I am convinced that all nurses need a working knowledge of the normal functioning of the human body. It is only when we understand the normal that the abnormal pathological situation makes any sense. If we can understand how the body goes wrong then it often becomes obvious what needs to be done to treat the disorder. So physiology and pathophysiology can both be used to inform our clinical interventions and provide us with rationales for care. This inevitably allows us to be more accountable in our practice and become more informed and knowledgeable practitioners.

I originally wrote these notes as a revision guide for my students and because they proved useful I decided to expand and publish them. The aim is to keep the text concise but to explain the physiology and necessary basic science in a way that is easy to understand. Diagrams are an important part of this philosophy. When I first discussed this book with the publisher we thought about getting the diagrams professionally drawn, but we decided that rather than produce beautiful pictures I would draw the diagrams myself just as I draw them for my students. If the diagrams are kept simple in this way they may be learned too – this takes practice but in the end it really helps us to understand the physiology. You may also find it helpful to colour some of the diagrams.

Physiology is not easy to learn, the terminology alone can be like learning a foreign language, but if you stick at it, both you and your patients will benefit for the rest of your career.

John Campbell
August 2002

CHAPTER 1

Cells, tissues and bodies

Introduction

Before we get down to some really interesting physiology it may be useful to define a few terms. Physiology is the study of the normal function of a biological system, in this case the human body. Anatomy is the study of normal structure. Inevitably, in order to understand physiology we must also learn some anatomy. Histology is the study of tissues and cytology the study of cells. Biochemistry is the study of the chemistry of living things, mostly the chemistry of the cell. Psychology studies the normal processes of the mind.

Pathology is the study of abnormal anatomy, and pathophysiology often means the study of abnormal body function. Histopathology studies abnormalities found in tissues. Psychiatry is the study of the abnormal mind.

Cells, tissues and organization

The body is a remarkably complex structure that performs thousands of physiological functions. This means the structures of the body must be organized in a precise way to carry out these functions. The functional systems of the body, such as the nervous or digestive systems, are themselves made up of organs such as the brain or stomach. Organs, in turn, are composed of precise arrangements of tissues. A tissue is a group of similar cells, often with associated additional structural material produced by the tissue cells. Cells that compose a particular tissue are themselves composed of smaller functional units called cell organelles. I think of organelles as the 'organs' of a cell. Cell organelles are made up of highly structured biomolecules such as proteins, carbohydrates and fats. Large

body
body systems
organs and large structures
groups of tissues
tissues
groups of cells and structural material
individual cells
cell organelles
large biomolecules
small organic molecules
atoms
electrons, neutrons, protons

Table 1.1 The body is very highly organized on a number of levels. This table indicates the hierarchy of this organization, starting with the largest and working down to the smallest.

biological molecules are made up of smaller organic compounds. (Organic simply means that the molecule contains some carbon.) The organic molecules are composed of structured arrangements of atoms, which are composed of protons, neutrons and electrons.

Cell organelles

The cell may be considered as the 'unit of life'. This means that many of the processes essential for life are carried out inside cells. Cytology is the term used to describe the study of cells. A single cell may be

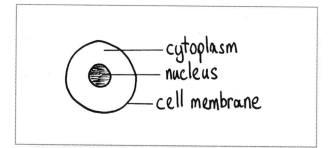

Diagram 1.1 Cell viewed under a light microscope with a magnification of about 300 times.

considered to be 'alive'. Some simple organisms such as the amoeba are composed of a single cell. However, in humans billions of cells combine to make up the body. As cells are only 5–10 micrometres (a micrometre is one thousandth of a millimetre) in size they can only be seen with the aid of microscopes. Under the light microscope a cell has a dark-staining central region called the nucleus, and the clear area surrounding this is referred to as cytoplasm. These components are all surrounded by a cell membrane that encloses the cell.

However, when cells are examined under the higher power of an electron microscope the organelles may be seen. These are sub-units or components of the cell. In the same way that a body is made up of organs, a cell is composed of organelles. Organelles are structures within the cytoplasm that perform specific functions. They are the functional units of a cell.

Cell membrane

This is a very thin membrane that surrounds the outside and marks the boundary of the cell. Cell membrane is composed of a combination of lipids, phosphates and proteins. Because the cell membrane appears to be in two layers it is referred to as a phospholipid bilayer. The external cell membrane compartmentalizes the cell and controls movement of fluid and other substances in and out. This regulatory function means the cell is able to control, to a degree, its own internal environment. Some of the proteins in the membrane act as receptor sites. These specialized areas allow the cell to recognize chemical messages from other cells or from endocrine glands. Once a receptor has detected the presence of a particular chemical messenger, this will initiate some physiological change within the cell.

Endoplasmic reticulum (ER)

This is an extensive network of channels distributed throughout the cytoplasm. Endoplasmic reticulum is itself bounded by membranes. The function of this extensive structure is to move materials around inside the cell, i.e. intracellular translocation. As different parts of the cell perform different functions, particular substances will be required in specific locations. In this sense the ER is analogous to a road or rail network, delivering raw materials and transporting away finished products. In addition, the ER provides support for the overall structure and shape of the cell.

The ribosomes are often associated with the ER. If an area of ER is associated with ribosomes it is described as rough ER; areas without associated ribosomes are termed smooth ER.

Ribosomes

These are small dark-staining organelles. They are often associated with rough endoplasmic reticulum but may be found anywhere in the cytoplasm. Rough endoplasmic reticulum is described as 'rough' because it is studded with ribosomes. Ribosomes receive genetic instructions from the DNA in the nucleus of the cell. They use this information to string together long chains of amino acids to form proteins. Amino acids are sub-units of proteins in the same way that bricks are sub-units of a wall. Ribosomes are therefore the site of protein synthesis – in essence they are little protein factories. Some of the synthesized proteins are used to form the structures of the individual cell and others are exported from the cell. It is logical that the ribosomes are usually associated with the ER so they can be supplied with raw materials and the finished proteins removed to where they are required.

Golgi

This is an arrangement of membranes which are responsible for the export of products from the cell. Products from the ER are transported to the Golgi where some further modifications sometimes take place. Once the fat- or protein-based product is ready, so-called secretory granules bud off the main Golgi complex and transport the material to the external cell membrane for export. For example, some cells in the digestive system secrete digestive enzymes in this way.

Mitochondria

All living cells must be able to produce energy to fuel physiological processes. When a cell is no longer able to produce energy it will quickly die. Mitochondria have an outer membrane and a highly enfolded inner membrane. The enfolded inner membrane provides a large surface area for the location of enzymes responsible for generation of energy within the cell. These enzymes produce energy by using oxygen to oxidize or 'burn' fuels such as glucose or fatty acids. The energy actually comes from breaking the chemical bonds which held together the fuel molecule. All of the fuel required for energy production derives from food and all of the oxygen from breathing. Mitochondria are therefore the site of all energy production and are sometimes referred to as the 'power-house' of the cell. Cyanide is such a fast-acting poison because it halts the process of energy production in mitochondria. Cells that use a lot of energy, such as those in muscles, have a lot of mitochondria in their cytoplasm whereas cells that need less energy, such as the cells that compose the skin, have fewer.

Lysosomes

Lysosomes are organelles that contain digestive enzymes such as lysozyme. For example, in white blood cells, when foreign material is ingested into the cell, lysosomes approach the foreign material and spill their digestive enzymes onto it, therefore digesting it. Lysosomes are therefore essential for the process of phagocytosis (this means cell eating, see page 118). Lysosomes may also burst to digest a cell that is unwanted by the body, in a form of cell suicide.

Cytosol

Cytosol is the fluid found in the cytoplasm of the cell. This contains some water and some larger molecules, the combination of which is

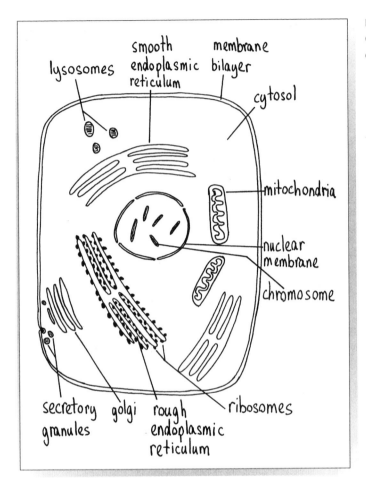

Diagram 1.2
Cell viewed under an electron microscope.

referred to as a colloid. Organelles are suspended within the cytosol. Much of the water in the body is located in cell cytosol.

Nucleus

The nucleus is located at the centre of the cell inside the cytoplasm. There is a separate membrane surrounding the nucleus referred to as the nuclear membrane. Within the nucleus are the chromosomes. All human cells (at least at some time in their lives) contain 46 of these bodies arranged in 23 pairs. Chromosomes contain the genes, which are the genetic information responsible for making and controlling the cell. This is why the nucleus is sometimes referred to as the 'control centre' of the cell.

Chromosomes

The term chromosome literally means coloured body. The chromosomes are composed of structural proteins and DNA (deoxyribonucleic acid). Genes are part of the chromosomes and are composed of DNA strands. Genes contain the genetic information to create the cell and therefore ultimately to generate the body.

Specialized cells

During growth and development cells specialize to form a particular function. Specialization is carried out under the genetic control of the genes. Different cells must have a specialized structure, which results in the production of many completely different types of cell. This process of cell specialization is referred to as differentiation. Specialized cells are required to form the different types of tissue needed to form the large structures and organs of the body. Different types of cells include nerve cells or neurones, muscle cells, liver cells, blood cells and epithelial cells. Each cell has a structure and function specific to the role that cell and tissue is required to perform in the body. Groups of similar cells compose tissues. Groups of tissues compose organs and groups of organs compose the systems of the body.

Cell reproduction

All cells are derived from parent cells which underwent a process of cell division. In this process one parent cell grows then divides into two daughter cells. There are only two forms of cell division, referred to as mitosis and meiosis.

Mitosis

Mitosis is simple cell division. A parent cell containing 46 chromosomes divides into two daughter cells each also containing 46 chromosomes. Because the daughter cells and the parent cell all contain the same number of chromosomes this form of cell division is sometimes referred to as conservation cell division (the number of chromosomes is conserved). This is the type of cell division that occurs when the body grows from the zygote (a fertilized egg), and it also occurs during wound healing. In addition, ongoing mitosis maintains the health of most body tissues. Because mitosis is the type of cell division that goes on in the body it is sometimes referred to as somatic cell division (soma means body).

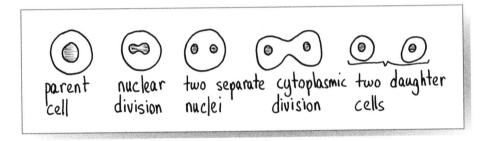

Diagram 1.3
The stages of mitosis in order.

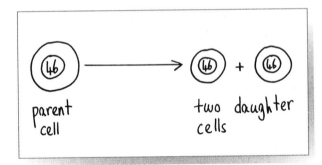

Diagram 1.4
The principle of conservation cell division. A parent cell with 46 chromosomes mitotically divides to produce two daughter cells also with 46 chromosomes. After formation the daughter cells will usually grow to be the same size as the parent.

Meiosis

The other form of cell division is called meiosis and is only used in the production of gametes, that is the sperm and ova. The function of sperm and ova is to fuse together, forming a fertilized cell. Such a fertilized cell is called a zygote. Once formed, a zygote undergoes repeated mitosis to form a new body. If the sperm and ovum each contained 46 chromosomes then the zygote, and hence the new baby, would contain 92 chromosomes. To prevent this increase in chromosome number the sperm and ovum are produced by meiosis, which is a reduction cell division. During meiosis the daughter cell (always a sperm or ovum) only receives one from each pair of chromosomes, leaving each sperm or ovum with 23 chromosomes. This means the zygote receives 23 chromosomes from the ovum and 23 from the sperm to give it a full complement of 46. Gametes are produced from germ cells which are located only in the testes and ovaries.

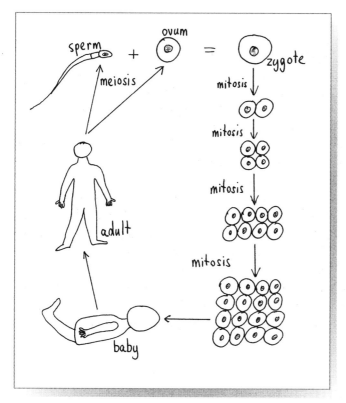

Diagram 1.5
Human life cycle. A male gamete fertilizes a female gamete to form a zygote. This divides by the process of mitosis to form the body. Growth then occurs. The next generation of gametes are formed by meiosis.

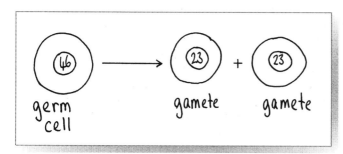

Diagram 1.6
Meiosis – the number of chromosomes is reduced from 46 to 23 per cell.

Diagram 1.7
During fertilization the sperm and the ova combine to produce a zygote with 46 chromosomes.

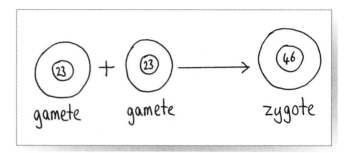

Cells and ageing

It seems that many cells have a limited number of times they can divide. Many of these permissible cell divisions take place between the formation of the zygote and the birth of the individual. This means in childhood and adult life only a limited number of further cell divisions are possible. When this number has occurred the cells are not capable of further divisions, which results in death of the cell line. If the number of viable cells in a tissue is reduced the result will be that the tissue as a whole deteriorates. As the body is composed of tissue, deterioration in tissues results in the changes in the body we associate with ageing. Ultimately tissues become so non-viable that they fail to perform essential physiological functions, possibly resulting in the death of the individual. For example, the tissues in the wall of a blood vessel may fail resulting in haemorrhage.

As cells age there may also be mistakes in the process of cell division. For example, mutation can occur as a result of a mistake in the production of a new chromosome or gene as the cell divides. The term mutation means a change in a gene or chromosome. This is analogous

Essential science

To measure how acid or alkaline a solution is, the pH scale is used. This is a scale that goes from 1 to 14. A strong acid such as hydrochloric acid has a pH of 1. Pure water is neutral – it is not acid or alkaline – so it has a pH of 7. A strong alkali such as sodium bicarbonate has a pH of 14. The lower the number under 7 the stronger the acid is, and the higher the number above 7 the stronger the alkali is.

to copying out a page of writing and misspelling or missing out some words. The accumulation of these errors in the genetic material of the cell may be one reason why many cancers are more common in older people than in younger people.

Another possible reason why cells age is given by free radical theory. A free radical is a very reactive form of oxygen that can oxidize and so damage cellular proteins. If the free radical attacks the DNA of the genes this may result in age-related changes and sometimes mutations leading to cancer. Free radicals are believed to be produced as a result of over-eating, exposure to radiation and exposure to polluting chemicals. Some vitamins and other components in fruit and vegetables inhibit the activity of free radicals and so may slow down cell ageing. This is one reason everyone is advised to eat at least five portions of fruit and vegetables per day.

As people age the rate of mitosis and tissue repair is also reduced as there is a generalized slowing in the rate of metabolic activity. This is one reason why wounds heal much faster in children than in elderly people.

Cells and enzymes

A cell is essentially a very complex chemical and molecular machine. A wide range of biochemistry is going on in the cell throughout its lifespan. In order to control the function of the cell it is therefore necessary to control the chemistry of the cell. All intracellular biochemistry is controlled by enzymes. An enzyme is a biochemical catalyst. A catalyst is a substance that facilitates or speeds up the rate of a chemical reaction without being used up in that reaction itself.

Each chemical process is catalysed by a specific enzyme. If this enzyme is absent, the particular chemical reaction cannot proceed. Each enzyme is synthesized from the genetic information carried by a specific gene. Enzymes are complex proteins formed into a particular shape; it is because of this complexity that they require specific conditions in order to function. For example they are specific to a particular temperature and pH range. This is one reason why people die if the body temperature is raised 6°C above normal, or the blood becomes acidotic. If body temperature rises beyond certain levels or there is a change in pH, the physical shape of some enzymes will be altered. As a result they will no longer be able to efficiently catalyse some cell biochemistry; this in turn will lead to interference with the physiology of the cell, and ultimately to cell death. (When reading physiology enzymes can always be recognized because their names end in '-ase'.)

Tissues

The study of tissues is referred to as histology and there are four principal types of tissue: epithelial, connective, muscle, and nervous.

Epithelial tissue

Epithelium describes any tissues that line or cover other structures. The internal and external surfaces of the body are lined with epithelial tissues. Epithelial tissues are composed of fairly tightly packed cells that are arranged on a sheet of fibrous tissue referred to as a basement membrane. The two main types of epithelium are simple and stratified.

A simple epithelium is one in which each individual cell is in contact with the basement membrane; this means simple epithelium is only one cell layer thick. There are different forms of simple epithelium, which are described according to the shape of the cells. Squamous epithelial cells are flat in shape and so form a very smooth surface. This is important in the lining of blood vessels, to allow a smooth flow of blood throughout the circulatory system. If the flow was turbulent clots might form. Cuboidal epithelial cells are cube-shaped cells and are found in nephrons and various endocrine glands. Columnar epithelial cells are rectangular or column-shaped and line such

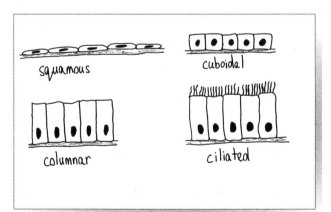

Diagram 1.8 Four forms of simple epithelium, squamous, cuboidal, columnar and ciliated. Each epithelial layer is one cell thick and is located on a basement membrane.

structures as the gastrointestinal tract. In the respiratory tract the columnar simple epithelium lining the airways has small hair-like structures called cilia. These help to waft mucus from the smaller airways towards the trachea. If cilia are present the lining is referred to as a ciliated epithelium.

A stratified epithelium is one in which some layers of cells are not in contact with the basement membrane so the epithelium consists of various strata (or layers) of cells. Different forms of stratified epithelium again may be made up of different types of cells; for example, stratified squamous epithelium consists of layers of flat-shaped cells. In a cuboidal epithelium there are several layers of cuboidal cells. In several stratified tissues the cells start off as cuboidal but become flattened by external pressures as they get nearer the surface.

Stratified epithelium is found lining surfaces which are subject to a degree of wear and tear. For example, the mouth is lined with stratified squamous epithelium. This means that during the relative trauma of chewing food, some of the surface cells may be sloughed away from the epithelium without disturbing the overall integrity of the lining. Similar epithelia line the vagina and oesophagus.

Some forms of stratified epithelium are keratinized and stratified. These occur on dry surfaces such as the skin that are subject to wear and tear. Keratin is a protein that is resistant to wear and is waterproof; it also acts as a barrier to the passage of bacteria.

Another form of stratified epithelium is referred to as transitional. This is composed of pear-shaped cells and is designed to allow the epithelium to stretch. It is found lining structures that need to alter their size such as the urinary bladder and urethra.

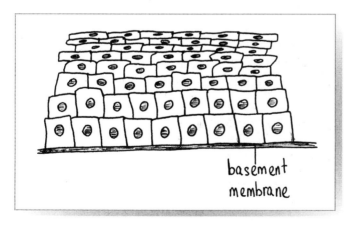

basement
membrane

Diagram 1.9 Stratified epithelium: several layers of cells on a basement membrane

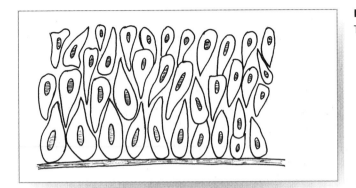

Diagram 1.10
Transitional epithelium.

Connective tissue

There are different types of connective tissues; usually they contain fewer cells than epithelium but contain more strong and elastic components to give the connective tissues firm structural properties. For example, white fibrous tissue is a strong connector composed of bundles of collagen fibres with a few fibroblasts included in the tissue. Collagen is a protein formed into bundles that have great tensile strength – they are analogous to ropes or cables and give tissue integrity and strength. This is why it is difficult to tear tissues. Fibroblasts are cells which produce the collagen protein.

The spaces between the cells and fibres in connective tissues are filled with ground substance, also sometimes referred to as the matrix. Ground substance is also produced by the fibroblasts and consists of water and glycoproteins. A glycoprotein is a large molecule made from a combination of protein and carbohydrate.

White fibrous tissue composes ligaments and periosteum (ligaments link bone to bone and periosteum surrounds the bones). As

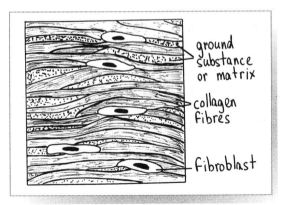

Diagram 1.11 Histology of white fibrous tissue.

ground substance or matrix

collagen fibres

fibroblast

ligaments link bones together, it is therefore white fibrous tissue that is largely responsible for holding the body together and keeping the bones in the correct positions relative to each other.

Elastic connective tissue is usually yellowish and stretchy; it is composed mostly of interlinking elastic fibres. Within the tissue are found fibroblasts; these are the cells which produce the elastic fibres. Like collagen, the elastic fibres are made up of a protein, but in elastic fibres the protein is called elastin. Elastin is found in such structures as the walls of blood vessels, lungs, the epiglottis and the ear lobes. The skin is also elastic due to the presence of elastic fibres. If you pinch up an area of skin and let it go, it quickly returns to its original shape because it is elastic.

In the case of blood vessels the elastic nature of the walls allows expansion when a pulse of blood is flowing through the vessel. However, when there is no pulse of blood the vessel wall will recoil becoming smaller again: this will maintain the blood pressure until the next pulse, smoothing out the blood flow. This effect maintains a more constant blood supply to tissues than an intermittent pulsed supply would provide. In the lungs the elastic nature of the tissue allows expansion during inspiration and aids the process of expiration by recoiling again. The recoiling of the air sacs increases the pressure of the air they contain and helps to 'blow' it out of the lungs.

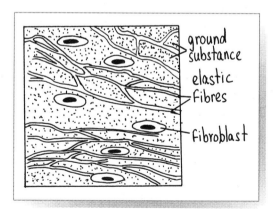

Diagram 1.12 Histology of elastic tissue.

Loose connective tissue is another common connector and is made up of a combination of elastic and collagen fibres. Again the tissue contains fibrocytes that produce the fibres. Loose connective tissue is found in areas of the body where tensile strength and elasticity are needed together. It is found underneath the skin and between muscle fibres where strength and elasticity are needed in combination. Some texts refer to loose connective tissue as areolar tissue.

Diagram 1.13 Histology of loose connective tissue.

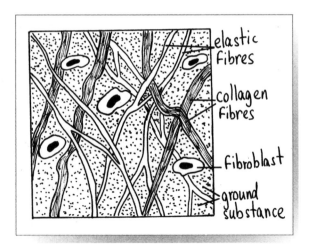

Adipose tissue is also classified as a connective tissue and composes the fat of the body. It is found under the skin where it acts as a padding to protect underlying structures. This is one reason it hurts so much when you knock your shin, as there is no fat lying over the bone to help protect it from trauma. Subcutaneous fat also gives insulation against the cold. Women store more fat under the skin than men, giving their limbs a more rounded appearance. Men store excess fat in the abdomen, giving the characteristic 'beer belly' appearance in obesity. Adipose tissue is also used to protect organs; for example the kidneys are embedded in a thick layer of fat. As fat is a fuel it also provides an energy reserve. Individual fat cells are called adipocytes and may take up or release fat depending on the food intake and metabolic requirements of the body. Each individual cell stores fat in a large central area called a vacuole. Adipose tissue also contains some collagen-based reticular fibres to give it structure and some strength. (Reticular or reticulum means to do with a network.)

Lymphoid tissue is also classified as a connective tissue. It is composed of a network of connective tissues termed a reticulum. These reticular fibres are very fine and composed mostly of collagen. Within this framework there are large numbers of immunologically active cells such as lymphocytes and monocytes. The main function of the lymphoid tissue is therefore to protect the body against the threat of infection. The lymph nodes, spleen, tonsils and part of the appendix are made out of lymphoid tissue.

Cartilage is a connective tissue that performs such functions as joining the ribs to the sternum and is also found between the vertebrae.

Diagram 1.14
Histology of adipose
tissue.

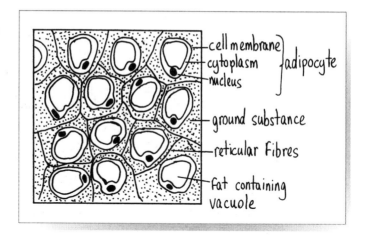

Articular cartilage lines the surfaces of joints to give a smooth, hard, low-friction surface between bones. Like other connective tissues, cartilage is composed mostly of connective tissue fibres made of collagen. The ground substance is hard but flexible, consisting of water, some collagen and some specialized large protein-based molecules. The cells in cartilage that produce the collagen and ground substance are also found within the tissue and are called chondrocytes.

Osseous tissue is described as a connective tissue and is another name for bone. Bone is hard in order to give the body a supportive framework. It also protects soft underlying structures such as the heart, lungs and brain. The basic structure of bone is similar to the other forms of connective tissue. It contains tough strong collagen fibres and cells that produce them. These cells responsible for bone production are called osteoblasts. The reason bone is so hard and rigid compared to other tissues is that the ground substance is mineralized with salts such as calcium phosphate.

Blood is also classified as a connective tissue and is discussed in Chapter 6.

Muscle tissue

Muscle is another classification of tissues. There are three main types of muscle: skeletal, cardiac, and smooth.

Skeletal muscle is sometimes referred to as striated and is attached to bones via tendons to allow movement of the skeleton. It is also sometimes called voluntary because it is under the control of our will.

Skeletal muscles are usually arranged in antagonistic pairs to allow movement in two or more directions. 'Antagonistic' means they are set in opposition to each other in order to bring about opposite movements. So, if you want to extend your arm the triceps muscle contracts; however, to fold the arm up the biceps muscle contracts. This arrangement is required because muscles can only contract – they cannot actively elongate themselves.

Skeletal muscle cells are unusual in that they contain many nuclei. The cells form long, striated structures termed fibres. 'Striated' means striped but these striations can only be seen using a microscope. Within the muscle fibres, i.e. inside the muscle cells, are arrangements of specialized contractile proteins. These proteins have the ability to reduce their length and so cause the muscle to contract. Contractile proteins comprise very small structures referred to as myofibrils ('myo' is the prefix that refers to muscle). The energy required for the contraction of the myofibrils is produced by mitochondria also located in the muscle cells. Muscle fibres are held together by connective tissue that continues on to form tendons at the end of the muscle.

Diagram 1.15 Skeletal muscle tissue.
(i) This shows a single muscle fibre with alternating dark and light bands; there are multiple nuclei.
(ii) A group of muscle fibres grouped together to form a muscle.

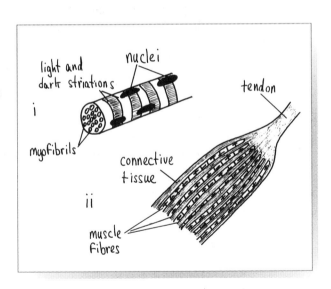

Cardiac muscle is only found in the heart and composes the myocardium, which is the middle muscular layer. The myocardium powers the contractions of the heart. Like skeletal muscle it is also somewhat striated in appearance. Because the cardiac muscle is not under direct control of the will it is a form of involuntary muscle. Individual cardiac muscle cells link up with each other to form networks throughout the tissue. These interconnections allow electrical impulses to travel across the tissue. This is important as the muscle is stimulated to contract by an electrical signal. Cardiac muscle is able to rhythmically contract about 70 times per minute for a full lifetime – this may be in excess of 2.8 billion (thousand million) individual contractions.

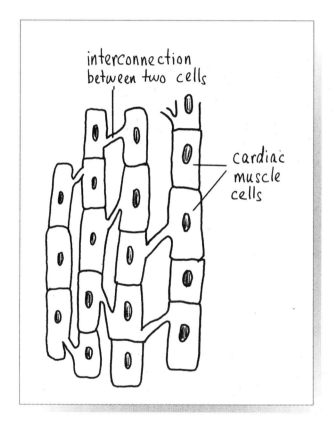

Diagram 1.16 Cardiac muscle tissue. Individual cells are interconnected.

Smooth muscle is not striated and is found in places like the walls of hollow structures, for example blood vessels, the stomach, the intestine and the bladder. It is usually involuntary, under the control of the autonomic (i.e. automatically controlled) nervous system. Smooth muscle contracts more slowly than striated muscle but it may contract very powerfully. For example, the myometrium composes the middle layer of the uterus and is composed mostly of smooth muscle; this is able to generate a force of contraction sufficient to deliver a baby through the birth canal during delivery. Often smooth muscle contractions are sustained and rhythmic in nature. The individual cells are long and tapered at the ends, and held together by connective tissue. Like striated muscles they contain contractile proteins but these are not arranged in a way that gives rise to a striated appearance.

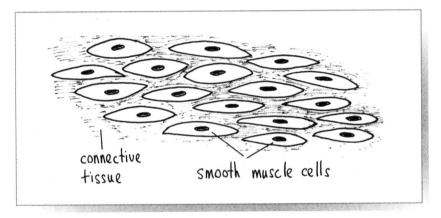

Diagram 1.17 Smooth muscle tissue. Individual muscle cells in a connective tissue.

Nervous tissue

Nervous tissue is composed of neurones or nerve cells. Some neurones carry nerve impulses from the central nervous system to muscles and are termed motor neurones. Motor means to do with movement; for example, a reduced motor function would mean a reduced ability to move. Nerve cells that carry information from sensory receptors into the central nervous system are called sensory neurones. These neurones are therefore essential for touch, taste, smell, sight and hearing. Nerve cells that connect other nerve cells together are sometimes called relay neurones. The nature and function of these cells are discussed more fully in Chapter 2.

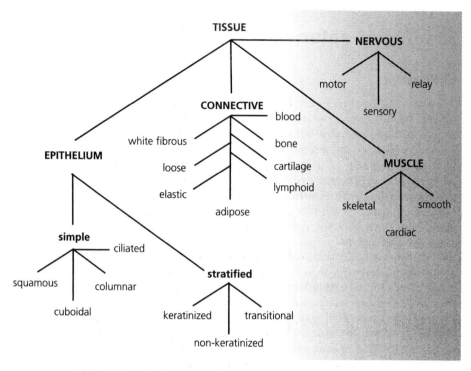

Table 1.2 Classification of body tissues.

Cells, tissues and fluids

In an average adult body there are approximately 40 litres of water, comprising around 57% of body weight. Most water, normally around 25 litres, is found inside the cells that comprise the body. Although in reality this water is located in billions of individual cells it is collectively referred to as the intracellular compartment. The rest of the fluid in the body is located outside the cells so is termed extracellular fluid. Total blood volume in an adult is usually 5 litres, which is located in the heart and various blood vessels, a space collectively referred to as the vascular compartment. This leaves approximately 10 litres of extracellular fluid which is located in the tissues. This tissue or interstitial fluid is located in the interstitial compartment, which in reality is in all of the tissue spaces of the body. This compartmentalization of body fluids is important for a number of physiological reasons, but we need to cover some science first.

Essential science

Diffusion

This can be defined as the process whereby liquids or gases of different concentrations mix up with each other when they are brought into contact, until their concentrations are equal throughout. For example, if you take a glass of clear water and put in a drop of ink, at first you will have an inky area while the rest of the water is still clear. However, over time, even if you do not stir it up, the whole glass will become inky as the ink molecules mix up with the rest of the water molecules in the glass.

This happens because the water and ink possess some heat energy. In a hot object the molecules are vibrating – in fact, the hotter the substance the more vigorously the molecules will be vibrating. This is the difference between a hot and a cold substance – in the hot the molecules are vibrating more energetically than in the cold. The result of this molecular movement is that the ink and water molecules vibrate into each other and end up mixing in together until their distribution is equal throughout the particular medium. The hotter the water, the more rapidly the process of diffusion will take place. Because diffusion requires the molecules to be able to move relative to each other the process can only take place in fluids, (gases and liquids are both defined as fluids). This principle of molecular vibration and heat is referred to as kinetic theory. Kinetic means to do with movement.

Diffusion is an essential physical process for numerous physiological processes. For example the concentration of oxygen in the air sacks of the lungs is higher than in the blood that is pumped to the lungs. Diffusion occurs in an attempt to make the concentration of oxygen equal in the air and in the blood. This results in the movement of oxygen from air into the blood. If this process were to suddenly stop we would die within a few minutes.

The rate at which diffusion occur depends on several factors, which include temperature, size and concentration of the particular molecules, pressure and the area over which diffusion is free to occur.

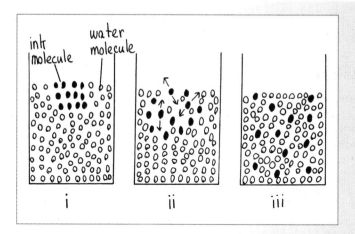

Diagram 1.18 The process of diffusion.

(i) Ink molecules are introduced into a glass of warm water.

(ii) Because the ink and water molecules are vibrating there are random collisions resulting in a mixing of the two fluids (only the vibration of three ink molecules is illustrated).

(iii) After a period of time and many random collisions the ink is equally distributed throughout the water.

Osmosis

Diffusion can occur in any fluid with any molecule that is soluble. However, osmosis is a special case of diffusion. It is the passage of water across a semi-permeable membrane under the influence of osmotic pressure. In physiology, osmosis only applies to the movement of water across biological membranes. A semi-permeable membrane will allow the free passage of water molecules but will restrict the movement of other molecules. In theory, if a membrane were fully permeable, it would allow the free passage of all molecules.

A useful way to learn about osmosis is to have a solution of pure water on one side of a semi-permeable membrane with a sugar solution on the other. The membrane will allow the passage of water molecules but will not be permeable to the sugar, because it is only semi-permeable. The process of diffusion means

that the water will diffuse through the membrane until the concentration of water molecules is equal on both sides. Despite this the sugar molecules will still only be on one side of the membrane. Because the sugar molecules take up space in the sugar solution the result is that there is a net movement of water molecules from the pure water side of the membrane to the sugar solution side of the membrane. It is this movement of water across the membrane that is referred to as osmosis. So water will diffuse from a watery solution to a less watery solution, i.e. osmosis waters things down.

Osmosis explains why we give saline and not pure water in intravenous infusions. If infusions contained

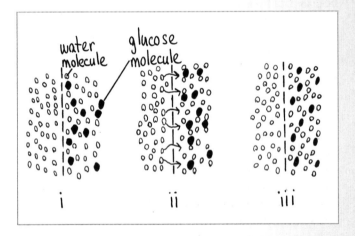

Diagram 1.19 The process of osmosis.
(i) Pure water and a glucose solution are separated by a semi-permeable membrane.
(ii) The water molecules are able to diffuse through the membrane because they are small, but the larger glucose molecules can not get through.
(iii) After a period of time the number of water molecules on both sides of the membrane will be the same. This means there has been a net movement of water into the sugar solution. In effect, the sugar solution has been watered down.

(Hint – try counting up the number of water molecules on both sides of the membrane in each diagram.)

pure water this would reduce the osmolarity of the blood and alter the osmotic balance between the plasma and the cytoplasm of red blood cells. This would mean that water from the diluted plasma would diffuse into the red cells and blow them up with water. This could result in some of the red cells bursting like over-filled balloons – this would lead to many pathological problems.

Importance of fluid compartmentalization

If you go out for a long walk on a hot day you could lose a litre or more of fluid as sweat. If you then lose your way home you could lose a further litre. This will mean you become thirsty but you will not die. Sweat is produced from water in the plasma by sweat glands. This means that during your walk, 2 litres of fluid was removed from the 5 litres of blood circulating in the body. If you lose 2 litres of blood in haemorrhage death can be the result; at the end of the walk, however, your blood pressure and blood volumes will still be normal. This means that the fluid in the blood has been replaced despite the fact you did not have access to a drink.

Blood contains large protein molecules called plasma proteins. These molecules give the blood its osmolarity, i.e. they make it osmotic so water will diffuse into it. When water is lost from the blood to produce sweat there is less water left so blood osmolarity increases as the blood becomes more concentrated and less watery. The result of this is that water diffuses through the semi-permeable membranes of the capillaries from the tissue fluid by the process of osmosis. This movement of water returns the blood volume to normal. However, if more water is sucked from the tissue fluid into the blood, the tissue fluid will, in turn, also become more osmotic. This will result in water moving from the intracellular compartment through the semi-permeable membranes of the cells into the interstitial compartment to maintain tissue fluid volumes. Tissue fluid does not contain proteins like plasma but osmolarity is generated by the presence of sodium (remember salt is sodium chloride).

So the compartmentalization of body fluids means there is a large fluid reserve to maintain blood volumes during periods of water loss when drinks are not available. Blood volumes will only be reduced when dehydration is severe.

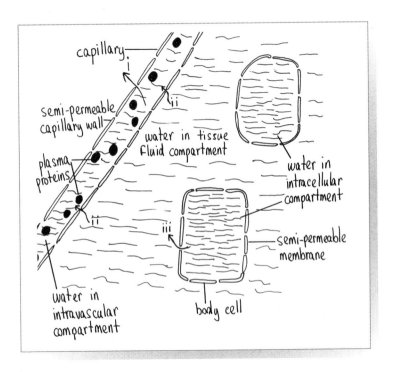

Diagram 1.20 Compartmentalization and osmotic movement of body fluids.
(i) When water is lost from the blood the osmolarity of intravascular fluid increases.
(ii) This results in water being osmotically sucked into the blood from the interstitial (or tissue) compartment.
(iii) As the osmolarity of the tissue fluid increases water diffuses out of the intracellular compartment by osmosis into the tissue fluid.

Whole body structure

Body cavities

Most of the organs of the body are contained in closed cavities. The cranial cavity is located inside the skull and houses the brain. This cavity is continuous with the vertebral cavity; this is inside the vertebral column and contains the spinal cord and some other large nerves. The thoracic cavity is located in the thorax or chest. At the back of the thoracic cavity are the 12 thoracic vertebrae, and the rest is surrounded by the ribs. This well-protected cavity contains the heart and lungs as well as the main airway and several major blood vessels. The bottom border of the thoracic cavity is marked by a domed sheet of muscle called the diaphragm.

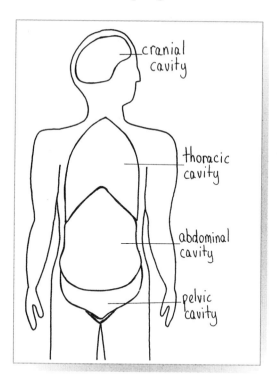

Diagram 1.21

The principal closed body cavities.

Below the diaphragm is the abdominal cavity. Behind this cavity are the large bones of the lumber vertebrae; most of the cavity is surrounded by sheets of muscle. An upper area is also protected by the lower ribs. Most of the digestive organs are found in the abdomen, as well as the liver, spleen and kidneys. Surrounding the abdominal cavity is a layer of connective tissue called the peritoneum. Below the peritoneum is the pelvic cavity, which is largely surrounded by the bones of the pelvis. The pelvis contains the bladder and reproductive organs. The testes are kept outside the pelvic cavity to keep them cool (sperm prefers temperatures of about 35°C).

CHAPTER 2

The nervous system

Introduction

The nervous system is an internal communication system allowing for rapid transport of messages within the body. This includes perception, processing of information and control of responses. Anatomically the nervous system may be divided into the central nervous system (CNS) and the peripheral nervous system (PNS). The CNS consists of the brain and spinal cord, and the PNS consists of all of the other nervous tissue in the body such as the nerves going to and from the spinal cord and the nerves in the limbs.

Nerve cells

The nervous system is composed of billions (thousand of millions) of individual specialized nerve cells referred to as neurones. These cells interconnect with other nerve cells to form networks that perform specific functions. Like any other cell, neurones are surrounded by a membrane and contain cytoplasmic organelles and a nucleus. There are different types of neurones that perform various functions, for example motor, sensory and relay neurones.

Motor neurones

'Motor' means 'to do with movement'. When we decide we want to move part of the body a motor neurone in the brain will generate a nerve impulse. The same neurone will then carry this message out and away from the central nervous system into the periphery where it will initiate the activity.

The nerve impulse is electrical in nature and is generated in the cell body. This is an enlarged area of the cell that contains the nucleus and most of the cell organelles. From here the impulse travels away, along a fibre of the motor neurone called an axon. Any nerve fibre that carries information (in the form of a electrical nerve impulse) away from a cell body is defined as an axon.

There are also dendrites connected to the motor neurone cell body. A dendrite is defined as any fibre that carries information towards a cell body. Typically a motor neurone consists of short dendrites conveying information towards the cell body and a longer axon carrying information away. Nerve fibres are essentially long thin projections of the cytoplasm. Despite being very thin, nerve fibres can be very long; for example, some motor neurone axons originate in the spinal cord and run the full length of the legs into the feet.

Because motor neurones initiate movement they often connect to skeletal muscles. When the axon approaches the muscle it supplies, the axon divides into a number of smaller fibres that end in specialized structures called the synaptic end bulbs. These bulbs are responsible for conveying the impulse from the axon to the muscle. The muscle will only contract when it is stimulated to do so by the nerve impulse. Because motor neurones carry impulses out from the CNS they are sometimes referred to as efferent neurones (I remember this by 'E is for Exit').

The importance of motor neurones is clearly seen in motor neurone disease, in which motor neurones progressively die. This results in increasing paralysis. Because it is only the motor neurones that die in this disease, sensation is not affected at all.

When we want to move a muscle, a nerve impulse is generated in the cell body which is located in the motor cortex of the brain. This is the area of the brain that initiates movement of the skeletal muscles. Nerve fibres from the motor cortex pass through the brain in a pathway called the internal capsule. They then cross over to the opposite side of the body at the level of the lower brain stem, before passing down the spinal cord. At the correct level in the spinal cord the first motor neurone connects with a second motor neurone via a small gap referred to as a synapse. This second motor neurone carries impulses from the spinal cord to the appropriate muscle. All of the motor neurones leave the spinal cord from the front; the pathway they take is referred to as the anterior nerve root.

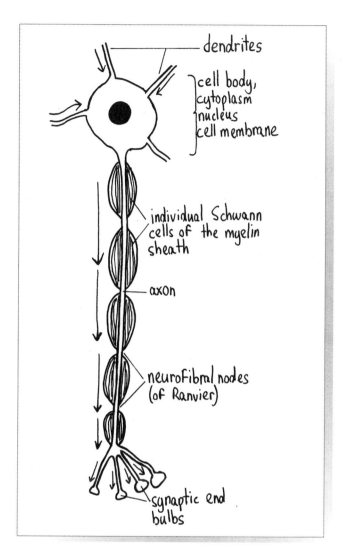

dendrites

cell body,
cytoplasm
nucleus
cell membrane

individual Schwann
cells of the myelin
sheath

axon

neurofibral nodes
(of Ranvier)

synaptic end
bulbs

Diagram 2.1
A motor neurone.
The arrows indicate the
direction of the nerve
impulse. Note the
dendrites carry the
impulse towards the cell
body and the axon carries
the impulse away.

Sensory neurones

Sensory neurones carry sensations from the environment to the sensory cortex in the brain. This is the area of the brain that allows us to detect the presence and location of sensation from the body. Stimuli from all five senses are transmitted via sensory neurones. In sensory neurones the nervous impulse is generated not in the cell body but in a peripheral sensory receptor. This is a specialized structure designed to detect a particular sensation, for example touch in the fingertips. When a sensation is detected the receptors generate a nerve impulse that represents the external stimulus. From the sensory receptor the impulse is transmitted along the dendrite of the sensory neurone to the cell body. This first fibre, between the receptor and the cell body, is referred to as a dendrite because it carries information towards the cell body.

From the cell body, an impulse is carried into the spinal cord via the axon of a sensory neurone. After entering the spinal cord the impulse travels upwards, towards the brain, in an ascending sensory pathway. At the level of the medulla, the first sensory neurone synapses with a second neurone. (The medulla is correctly termed the medulla oblongata.) This second neurone then crosses over to the opposite side of the medulla. An impulse then passes up through the brain stem to the thalamus where the second sensory neurone synapses with a third. The thalamus is an area of the brain with many interconnections, communicating between the brain and spinal cord. (I think of the thalamus as a relay station.) It is the third sensory neurone that carries the impulse into the sensory cortex of the brain where it is experienced as sensation.

The arrival of a sensory stimulus in the sensory cortex generates the experience we call tactility or feeling. In this sense, ultimately, all sensation is generated by the brain. This means if I hit my thumb with a hammer, it feels to me like the pain is in my thumb. In fact the pain is experienced in the area of my sensory cortex that corresponds to my thumb.

Like motor neurones the fibres of the sensory neurone have a myelin sheath. Because sensory neurones carry information into the CNS they are sometimes referred to as afferent neurones.

Sensory neurones enter the cord from the back, via the posterior nerve root. All of the cell bodies of the sensory neurones, carrying information into the spinal cord at a particular level, are located in a group or cluster. This group of cell bodies is referred to as the posterior root ganglion. A ganglion is a cluster of cell bodies in the PNS. (If a group of cell bodies is found in a cluster in the CNS this is referred to as a nucleus.) On entering the spinal cord some sensory neurone axons synapse, and cross over to the opposite side and then travel up the spinal cord. Other sensory neurones, as discussed, do not cross over until the level of the brain stem. However, the end result is always that sensation from the right side of the body is experienced in the left side of the brain and sensation from the left side of the body is experienced in the right side of the brain. The reason for this cross-over is currently unclear.

Diagram 2.2

A sensory neurone.

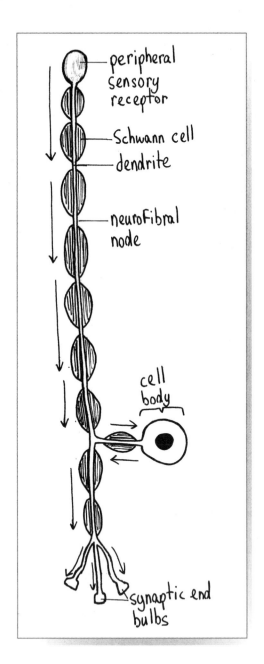

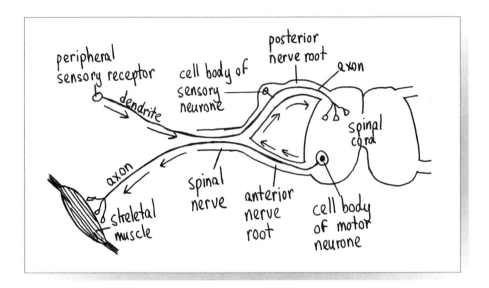

Diagram 2.3 Transverse section of the spinal cord showing motor and sensory nerve roots. Again the arrows illustrate the direction the nerve impulses follow. The motor neurone receives impulses from a descending neurone coming down from the brain and the sensory neurone connects to an ascending neurone that carries the impulse up towards the brain. (Note only the nerve roots on the right side of the body are illustrated.)

The motor and sensory nerve fibres leave and enter the spinal cord separately. However, a short distance away from the cord they join to form a single spinal nerve.

Relay neurones

In addition to motor and sensory neurones there are other nerve cells that connect these together. Sometimes referred to as relay neurones, they relay an impulse from one neurone to another. More correctly they are termed interneurones or association neurones. These interneurones also consist of a cell body with associated nerve fibres.

Myelin

Nerve cells and fibres are of course microscopic. A group of nerve fibres will run together in a bundle forming a macroscopic structure referred to a nerve. Macroscopic means large as opposed to microscopic which means small. As a nerve consists of many nerve fibres, carrying electrical nerve impulses, there is a risk that the impulses will jump from one fibre to another forming a short circuit. In order to prevent this, each individual nerve fibre is insulated. This insulation is provided by a specialized form of cell. In the PNS these specialized insulating cells are referred to as Schwann cells which wrap themselves around the nerve fibres. Schwann cells are composed of an insulating fatty material called myelin that forms a sheath around the nerve fibres. The myelin sheath is therefore like the PVC insulation that surrounds a copper wire. However, unlike an electrical insulator there are small gaps between the Schwann cells called the neurofibral nodes (also called the nodes of Ranvier).

In addition to insulating the nerve fibres, myelin increases the speed at which the impulse passes along the fibre (i.e. it increases the rate of neuronal transmission). Myelin also protects the nerve fibres from damage and helps with their nourishment. The vital function of the myelin sheath is illustrated in the condition of multiple sclerosis where there is a loss of myelin in the CNS.

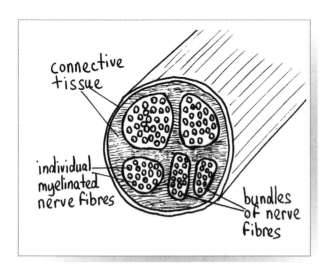

Diagram 2.4 Cross-section of a nerve composed of possibly thousands of nerve fibres in combination with fibrous tissue.

Essential science

In order to understand the nature of a nerve impulse it is necessary to understand how atoms can be electrically charged.

Atoms

An atom is made up of protons and neutrons that are closely grouped together in the atomic nucleus. Surrounding this core are orbiting electrons. These three sub-atomic particles possess mass and have a charge that may be positive, negative or neutral. The charge is electrical in nature. Protons carry a positive charge of +1 and electrons have a negative charge of –1. Neutrons are electrically neutral. Atoms are always electrically neutral. This means they must have the same number of positive protons as negative electrons. In this way, all of the negative and positive charges will cancel out to make the atom electrically neutral overall.

Ions

If an atom loses an electron it will lose one of its negative charges. This will mean there is one more positive charge than negative charges. This will give the atom an overall charge of +1. When an atom has an electrical charge it is no longer referred to as an atom but an ion. If an atom loses two electrons it will lose two negative charges and so will become an ion with an overall charge of +2. Conversely if an atom gains an electron it will become an ion with a charge of negative one and if it gains two electrons it will become an ion with a charge of –2.

Diagram 2.5

Atoms and ions.

(i) A sodium atom containing 11 protons and 11 electrons is electrically neutral.

(ii) A sodium ion forms when the atom loses an electron and so has an overall charge of +1.

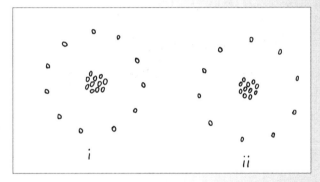

Neuronal transmission

We have already mentioned that a nerve impulse is electrical. This electrical charge is generated by the relative distribution of ions on both sides of the cell membrane. If there are more negative ions inside the cell with relatively more positive ions outside, the overall charge will also be negative on the inside and positive on the outside. This state is sometimes referred to as the resting potential. This is the electrical condition that a nerve fibre will be in when there is no nerve impulse passing a particular point. Because in this situation there is a negative pole inside and a positive pole on the outside, the cell is described as being polarized. These are the same as the poles of a battery, one of which is negative and the other positive.

However, when a nerve impulse is passing a point on a nerve fibre, the polarity across the cell membrane reverses. There is a change in the permeability of the membrane surrounding the nerve fibre. This in turn allows a change in the relative distribution of positive and negative ions on the two sides of the cell membrane. The result is that the inside becomes positive and the outside negative. This reversal of polarity is referred to as depolarization. After the nerve impulse has passed, the polarity reverts back to being negative inside and positive outside. The process by which resting polarity is restored is termed repolarization. When a nerve impulse is passing along a nerve fibre there is a wave of depolarization that passes along. It is this electrical wave that constitutes the nerve impulse. So the changes in polarity are brought about by changes in the relative distribution and concentration of ions. These concentrations may change because ions are able to pass through the cell membrane in specialized small gaps called ion channels.

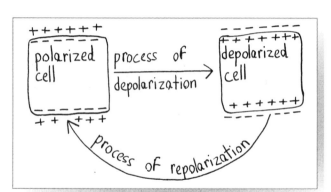

Diagram 2.6 An area of nerve fibre is polarized at rest. When the nerve impulse is passing it becomes depolarized; after the impulse has passed repolarization occurs.

Diagram 2.7 This shows the same length of nerve fibre as a nerve impulse passes along; the three illustrations are a fraction of a second apart.

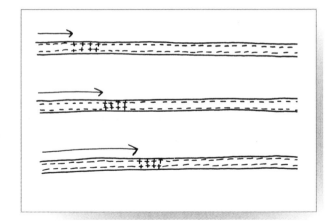

Speed of a nerve impulse

The speed at which a nervous impulse travels varies, depending on the type of neurone involved. Wider diameter fibres transmit impulses faster than narrow fibres. However, in humans the main factor influencing the rate of transmission is the presence of the myelin sheath. Myelinated fibres transmit the impulse quickly because the impulse does not need to travel along the full length of the fibre but is able to 'bounce' from one neurofibral node to the next. This is referred to a saltatory transmission. In unmyelinated fibres the speed of transmission may be as slow as 0.5 metres per second; however, in some myelinated fibres the rate may be over 100 metres per second.

Diagram 2.8 Saltatory or 'bouncing' transmission. This is analogous to a flat stone skimming over the surface of a lake – it hits the water then bounces further on.

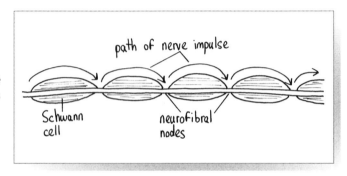

The synapse

There are very small gaps between individual nerve cells and between motor neurones and muscles: these gaps are called synaptic gaps. The gap is a physical space and the electrical nerve impulse is unable to jump across. The synapses are necessary to limit the propagation of an impulse around the nervous system. If all of the neurones were directly physically interconnected then any one nerve impulse would be propagated around the whole nervous system resulting in gross over-activity (which would probably result in continuous convulsions).

However, despite this need for electrical limitations, it is essential that nerve impulses can pass from one neurone to another when required. To allow this to happen the nerve fibre at one side of the gap releases a chemical called a chemical transmitter. This transmitter will then diffuse across the gap and generate a further electrical nervous impulse in the second neurone. Only the nerve fibre on one side of the synapse is able to secrete chemical transmitter. This means an impulse can travel from this first neurone to the second but not back in the other direction. The result is that synapses act as valves, only allowing one-way transmission of impulses.

The neurone before the gap is termed the pre-synaptic neurone and the one after the gap as the post-synaptic neurone. Just before the gap, the pre-synaptic neurone widens out into a structure called the synaptic end bulb. This contains mitochondria to provide energy for the function of the synapse. The bulb also contains vesicles of transmitter substances that have been previously synthesized by the neurone. When a nerve impulse arrives in the synaptic end bulb it causes some secretory vesicles to fuse with the pre-synaptic membrane releasing some chemical transmitter into the gap. After diffusing across the gap these transmitter molecules bind on to specific receptor sites on the post-synaptic membrane. Binding of transmitter into the receptor site activates the site. When enough of these receptor sites are activated by the chemical transmitter a further electrical impulse is generated in the post-synaptic neurone.

If an impulse should arrive at the synapse via the post-synaptic neurone it will not be able to cross the gap and so will terminate. So, a nerve impulse is electrical when travelling along nerve fibres and chemical when travelling across a synaptic gap. A synapse may occur between two nerve fibres or between a nerve fibre and a cell body.

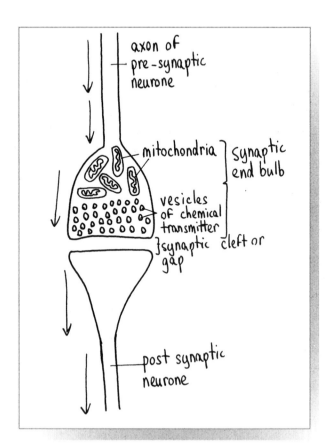

axon of
pre-synaptic
neurone

mitochondria] synaptic
] end bulb

vesicles
of chemical
transmitter
}synaptic cleft or
gap

post synaptic
neurone

Diagram 2.9 The synapse.
Arrows illustrate the
direction of the impulse.

The connection between the synaptic end bulb of a motor neurone and a muscle is also via a synapse. Because this junction connects
a nerve to a muscle it is referred to as a neuromuscular junction. As in
a nerve-to-nerve connection, chemical transmitter is released, diffuses
across the gap and binds onto specific receptor sites. When sufficient
of the receptor sites are activated by the binding of transmitter, the
muscle will be stimulated to contract. The surface of the muscle where
the receptor sites are located is termed the motor end plate.

Chemical transmitters

There are a wide range of chemical transmitter molecules used in the
nervous system. Two common transmitters are acetylcholine and
noradrenalin (the Americans call this norepinephrine). Acetylcholine

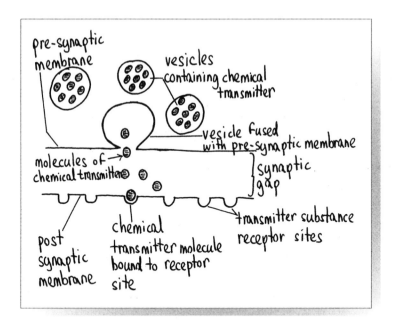

Diagram 2.10 This diagram illustrates the synapse at greater magnification. Transmitter molecules of a particular shape are able to fit into, and so activate, specific receptor sites on the post-synaptic membrane.

Diagram 2.11
A neuromuscular
junction.

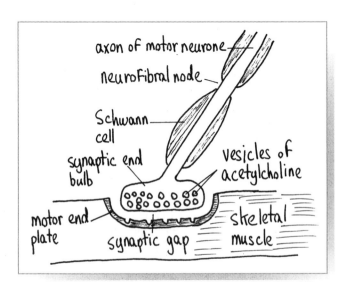

is also the neuromuscular transmitter molecule. Once the chemical transmitter has activated the post-synaptic membrane it has to be removed. If this is not done there will be continued stimulation. Some of the transmitter simply diffuses away into the tissue fluid. However, some is actively reabsorbed by the pre-synaptic neurone for recycling. In addition, in the case of acetylcholine, the molecule is broken down and inactivated by a tissue enzyme called acetylcholinesterase.

There are a large number of different transmitter molecules found in the CNS with a wide variety of functions. For example, there is a transmitter called GABA that inhibits the activity of many neurones. If the levels of GABA are increased, the individual feels relaxed and at ease. Anti-anxiety drugs often work by increasing GABA activity. Another transmitter is dopamine – this is vital for normal control of movement, and its deficiency causes Parkinson's disease. In other parts of the brain dopamine causes the person to experience pleasure. Levels of dopamine are increased by many drugs that people take for their enjoyable effects, such as alcohol or cocaine. Antidepressants work by increasing the amounts of serotonin by inhibiting pre-synaptic reuptake. This indicates that a feeling of depression is caused by low levels of serotonin. Endorphin is a transmitter molecule that reduces pain. Morphine-based drugs work because they activate endorphin receptor sites, simulating an endorphin effect.

When people artificially stimulate the levels of chemical transmitters by taking drugs the body often responds by producing less of its own. This is why many drugs have withdrawal or abstinence syndromes.

The reflex arc

Reflexes occur to protect the body from tissue damage; they are rapid involuntary actions. For example, the arm will suddenly be withdrawn if it touches a very hot object. A reflex arc describes an arrangement of three neurones that detect the stimulus and relay the information across the spinal cord to a motor neurone that will move an appropriate muscle.

The initial sensation is detected by peripheral sensory receptors and transmitted along the dendrite of a sensory neurone to the cell body. From the cell body it is then transmitted along the axon of the sensory neurone. This fibre then goes into the spinal cord where it synapses with a relay neurone. The relay neurone will carry the impulse across the spinal cord from the back, where the sensory neurones enter, to the front where the motor neurones leave. This relay neurone then synapses with the cell body of a motor neurone that carries the impulse away from the spinal cord to the appropriate muscle, which is innervated to contract, withdrawing the hand away from the hot object.

In addition an ascending neurone carries the information up the spinal cord to inform the brain of what has happened. This means that the reflex can occur before the brain becomes aware there is a problem. This saves a lot of time: if the message had to go up to the brain, from where a further message had to be sent down to the muscle, there would be a time delay during which injury could occur. There are many other examples of reflexes, including the eyelash and gag reflexes.

Sensory neurones always approach the spinal cord from the back and the motor neurones always leave the spinal cord from the front. The nerve containing the sensory neurones that pass into the spinal cord is termed the posterior root and the one containing motor neurones the anterior root. Posterior always means towards the back and anterior towards the front.

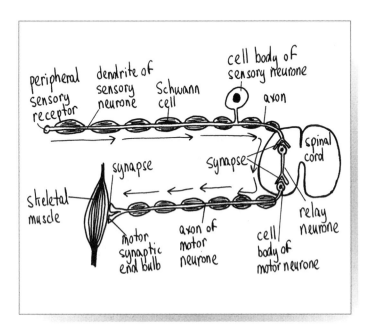

Diagram 2.12
A reflex arc.

The brain

The human brain is the most complicated known structure in the universe. A brain is composed of grey and white matter; grey matter is mostly nerve cells, and white matter is mostly nerve fibres. It is useful to think of the brain as consisting of four basic areas. These are the cerebrum, cerebellum, diencephalon and brain stem.

Diagram 2.13 Four main areas in the brain.

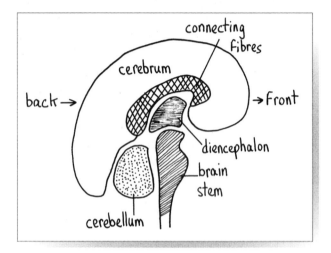

Cerebrum

The cerebrum is the largest part of the brain and is made up of the left and right cerebral hemispheres. These two sides of the brain are connected by a large number of connecting fibres. The outer layer of the cerebrum is called the cerebral cortex. This layer is folded to give a large surface area. Each of the hemispheres is composed of four lobes: these are the frontal, parietal, temporal and occipital lobes.

The motor area of the brain is located in the frontal lobes. This area contains the cell bodies of the motor neurones. Speech is also generated in an area of the frontal lobe just underneath the motor cortex. Frontal areas of the brain are concerned with various functions such as reasoning and abstract thinking. In addition, much of the personality and character seem to be generated in this area of the brain. If the frontal lobes are damaged the person become disinhibited, often severely.

The parietal lobe contains the sensory cortex. This is the area of the brain that collects information about the body generated in the

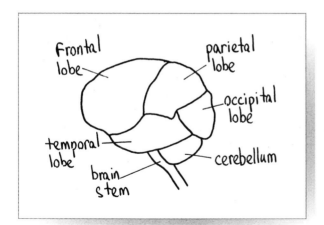

Diagram 2.14

Four main areas or lobes in the cerebrum (the brain stem and cerebellum are also identified).

peripheral sensory receptors and transmitted via sensory neurones. Different parts of the sensory cortex generate perception of sensation from different parts of the body. This area generates our positional sense so we know where various parts of the body are in space – this is why we can still clap hands with our eyes shut. The speech sensory area is also in the parietal lobe – this area allows us to understand language.

The auditory area – concerned with hearing – is in the temporal lobe, just underneath the sensory cortex. This lobe also contains the olfactory area, which generates the sense of smell from information received from the nose. The temporal lobe also seems to allow us to have religious experiences, and aids in the formation of emotions.

The occipital lobe is located at the back of the cerebrum and is the area where vision is generated. Nerve impulses arrive from the eye and the occipital lobe allows us to perceive these as vision.

While it is true that these specific lobes have many specific localized functions, it seems that much of the activity of the cerebral cortex is more diffuse. Processes such as thinking, memory and reasoning can still carry on even if some localized areas of the cortex are damaged. The experience of consciousness is also probably a diffuse product of the function of the cerebrum. This is why we measure Glasgow Coma Scales in head injuries. If the cortex is being compressed by rising pressure within the skull there will be a generalized reduction of cortical function, resulting in a corresponding reduction in the level of consciousness and so in GCS.

The cerebral cortex is particularly well developed in people compared to animals. It gives us the ability to function in groups, to relate to other people and to cooperate. If the activity of the cerebral cortex is reduced, then the social inhibitions that allow us to function in groups are inhibited. Alcohol causes loss of inhibitions by depressing the function of the cortex. This means that, while drunk, people may engage in behaviours that have social and personal consequences that they would not take part in if their cerebral cortex was functioning normally. Violent and sexual behaviour are the obvious examples.

Cerebellum

The cerebellum controls automatic learned functions such as writing, walking, making beds and riding a bike. Once these complex skills have been well learned the cerebellum can coordinate them, leaving the rest of higher parts of the brain free to think about something else. This is why we can make beds or drive a car while chatting about something more interesting. The cerebellum is also involved in functions such as balance, maintenance of posture, fine motor coordination and dexterity.

Diencephalon

This contains two structures: the thalamus and, below this, the hypothalamus. The thalamus is responsible for such apparently diverse functions as language, recent memory and emotion. It also acts as a relay centre, receiving information from the body via the spinal cord and relaying this on to appropriate areas of the brain. The hypothalamus is the main brain centre for regulation of the internal environment of the body, which means it controls several aspects of homeostasis. Among the parameters it regulates are body temperature, hunger, thirst, emotional balance, sexual behaviour and endocrine hormone homeostasis.

Brain stem

The brain stem acts as a connection between the spinal cord and the rest of the brain. Throughout the brain stem is a complex network of neurones called the reticular activating system: these generate consciousness. Although consciousness is generated in the brain stem it is probably mostly experienced in the cerebrum.

Anatomically, the brain stem is described in three areas. The upper region is the midbrain. This contains fibres to allow communication between the brain above and the body below. Below the midbrain is an area called the pons. Nerve fibres running through the pons are continuous with those of the midbrain above and medulla below. It also contains nuclei involved in motor and sensory innervation of the face in addition to areas which effect respiration.

The lower section of the brain stem is the medulla oblongata, often simply called the medulla. Again nerve fibres running through this area are continuous with the spinal cord below and the pons above. It is at the level of the medulla that many of the motor and sensory fibres cross over from left to right and visa versa. This is why if a person has a stroke that affects the right side of the brain the left side of the body is affected. Many vital nuclei are contained in the medulla oblongata. These include the respiratory centre, which controls breathing. Also in this region is the vasomotor centre, which controls the tone of blood vessels and helps to regulate blood pressure. There is also a cardiac centre, which influences the activity of the heart. It is because of this association of the brain stem with these vital physiological functions and consciousness that death is often now defined as death of the brain stem.

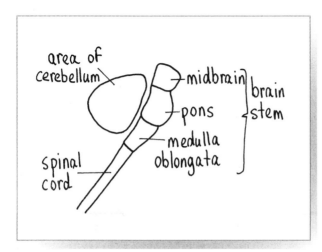

Diagram 2.15
The three areas of the brain stem.

Cranial nerves

These are the nerves that communicate directly with the brain without going via the spinal cord. There are 12 pairs of cranial nerves, usually numbered with Roman numerals. The cell bodies for these nerves are located in the brain, many originating from nuclei in the medulla oblongata. Some cranial nerves carry motor fibres, others sensory, and a few carry motor and sensory fibres. Sensory functions include sight, smell, hearing and sensation from the face, lips and teeth. Because these structures are physically above the level of the spinal cord it makes sense that they communicate with the brain directly. Cranial nerve motor functions include movement of the eyeball, control of the pupil, and movement of the tongue and facial muscles.

Cranial nerve control of the pupil explains why we check the response and diameter of the pupil in cases of head injury. The pupil is controlled by the third cranial nerve, which runs under the base of the brain. If this nerve is compressed by pressure from above it will not function properly, causing the pupil it controls to become sluggish and ultimately fixed in response to light.

Spinal cord

The spinal cord is the main communication route between the brain and body; in an adult it is about 45 cm in length. The meninges and cerebrospinal fluid (CSF) continue around and below the cord.

The outside of the cord is composed mostly of white matter, and an area in the centre is composed mostly of grey matter. As in the brain, the grey matter is mostly nerve cell bodies and white matter is the nerve fibres. In the spinal cord these nerve fibres carry the nerve impulses travelling between the brain and body. The spinal cord communicates with the body through 31 pairs of spinal nerves. These carry motor and sensory fibres. If there is a transverse injury to the cord the person will not be able to feel or move anything below the level of the lesion.

The spinal cord is anatomically described in sections, which are named according to the vertebrae in the region the cord is passing through. The top section is continuous with the medulla of the brain stem and passes through the neck; this is the cervical region. The second, thoracic region passes through the thorax. Thirdly, the lumbar region passes into the small of the back. In most people the spinal cord terminates between the level of the first and second lumbar vertebrae. This is why if a specimen of CSF is needed, the lumber puncture is normally performed below the third lumbar vertebra, to prevent accidental damage to the cord. Below the level of the second lumbar vertebrae, large spinal nerves form the lower lumbar, sacral and coccyx sections. As the spinal cord has terminated by this level these large nerves are no longer part of the spinal cord; they are collectively referred to as the cauda equina – Latin for 'horse's tail'.

Protection of the CNS

Nervous tissue is delicate and must be protected from trauma. To achieve this there are several layers of protection around the brain and spinal cord. The skull is surrounded by skin and subcutaneous tissue, which provide some cushioning effect against knocks. Hair may also provide a cushioning effect from outside forces. Under the subcutaneous tissue there is the periosteum and bone of the skull. The bone is strong and ridged and the skull forms a closed vault around the brain. The spinal cord is protected by the bony vertebrae.

Meninges

Under the bone there is a layer called the dura mater composed of tough fibrous tissue that supports and protects the brain and spinal cord. Underneath the dura mater is a web-like structure referred to as the arachnoid mater, which carries a lot of the blood vessels that supply blood to the brain. Underneath the arachnoid mater is the cerebrospinal fluid (CSF). This is contained in the space under the arachnoid mater, referred to as the subarachnoid space. In adults there is about 150 ml of this fluid surrounding the brain and cord. Underneath the cerebrospinal spinal fluid, lining the surface of the brain itself, is the pia mater. (Memory point – the CSF is at 'lunch time', between the morning and the afternoon, i.e. between the a.m. and the p.m.)

Collectively the dura, arachnoid and pia mater are called the meninges. Inflammation of the meninges causes meningitis. (I remember that the meninges PAD the brain – pia, arachnoid, dura.)

So the brain is protected from damage by hair, skin, subcutaneous tissue, bone, dura mater, arachnoid mater, pia mater and cerebrospinal fluid. The brain and spinal cord are essentially suspended in cerebrospinal fluid that acts as an excellent shock absorber. This prevents the brain from coming into contact with the inside of the skull every time the body is subjected to forces from outside.

Diagram 2.16
Protection of the
central nervous system
from damage.

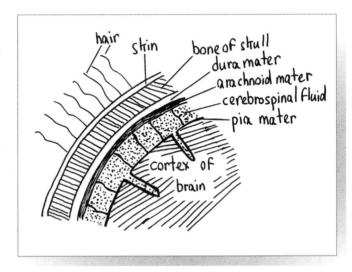

Blood brain barrier

The blood brain barrier is a physiological barrier between the blood supply to the brain and the brain interstitial fluid that bathes the neuronal cells themselves. This barrier is located in the capillary walls that carry blood to the brain tissue. Cells which form the walls of the brain capillaries are very tightly fitted together to prevent escape of certain drugs and toxins, which may otherwise get into the brain and poison it.

Autonomic nervous system

In physiological terms the nervous system can be divided into the voluntary nervous system – under the control of will – and the autonomic nervous system which functions automatically. The voluntary nervous system allows us to implement voluntary movements, for example, when we decide to move a hand or foot. The autonomic nervous system looks after the automatic functions controlled by the nervous system. The autonomic nervous system is itself subdivided into two sub-categories known as the sympathetic autonomic nervous system and the parasympathetic autonomic nervous system.

Sympathetic

The sympathetic nervous system prepares the body for 'fight or flight' – to escape from dangerous situations or to fight, if necessary. Sympathetic activity increases in an emergency, excitement and exercise (known as the 3 Es). Therefore it increases heart rate and the amount of blood pumped out per cardiac contraction (known as stroke volume); the combination of these factors increases cardiac output. This is why we can feel our hearts beating when we are anxious. It also increases respiratory rate and dilates the bronchial passages; these effects increase the amount of oxygen the lungs can absorb and the volume of carbon dioxide they can excrete. Again this prepares us for the vigorous exercise required to run or to fight.

Sympathetic innervation also causes dilatation of the blood vessels supplying skeletal muscles; this will allow them to exercise efficiently by increasing their supply of glucose and oxygen. However, because the blood volume is limited, the blood flow to other areas must be reduced. This is achieved by vasoconstriction of the blood vessels carrying blood to the skin and the gut. The vasoconstriction to the skin explains why someone may appear white when they are frightened. Reduced blood supply to the gut probably explains the feeling of 'butterflies' in the stomach when we are anxious. So reduced blood flow to the skin and gut leaves more blood to circulate around the heart, lungs and skeletal muscles. Sympathetic stimulation dilates the pupils of the eye to allow in more light so that the environment may be sensed and danger recognized. All of these effects make the body ready to take emergency action that will increase the chances of individual survival.

Parasympathetic

The parasympathetic nervous system usually has the opposite effect to the sympathetic. It reduces heart rate and stroke volume and also slows down the respiratory rate as well as constricting the bronchioles. This is appropriate when less air is required to go in and out of the lungs; if the airways remained wide open all the time, infection would be more likely. Vasodilatation increases the blood supply to the skin and the gut. Parasympathetic stimulation increases gut motility and stimulates the release of digestive enzymes to promote digestion. Vasoconstriction decreases the blood supply to skeletal muscles and the pupils constrict. The generally reduced level of activity facilitated by parasympathetic activity allows the body to conserve energy supplies.

So the parasympathetic nervous system is concerned with the more routine, low-key functioning of the body. It is the relative balance of innervation of the sympathetic and parasympathetic nervous system that maintains the body in a healthy physiological balance.

Repair

Neurones cannot divide to regenerate damaged nervous tissue. This means that damage to the brain or spinal cord after birth will usually result in a deficit of function. If the spinal cord is severed the nerve cells cannot divide to regenerate the lost tissues, so the person will be left paralysed for the rest of their lives. This is why it is vital to assume unconscious patients with head or neck injuries have cervical spinal damage until proved otherwise. When areas of the brain are killed the nerve cells will not be able to divide to repair the damage. In dementia there is a global loss of the cells of the cerebral cortex, which is why dementia is irreversible. When tumours arise in the nervous system they are caused by excessive mitosis of the neuroglial cells, not of the neurones. The neuroglial cells are supporting and structural cell types found in the nervous system.

Sleep

Sleep is marked by a reduced level of brain activity that reduces the level of consciousness. There is also diminished activity of skeletal muscles and a lowered metabolic rate. There are basically two types of sleep: rapid-eye-movement sleep (REM) and non-rapid-eye-movement sleep (NREM). Periods of REM sleep last for a few minutes to half an hour and alternate with NREM periods; dreaming occurs during REM sleep. The amount of sleep required by an individual changes throughout life from as much as 20 hours a day in infancy to as little as 6 hours a day in old age.

Possible reasons for sleep

Sleep allows the CNS to reduce its level of activity and so recuperate from the previous days activity. Dreaming may be necessary for the normal functioning of the CNS; some have suggested it is necessary for encoding learned information or for forgetting. People who have been deprived of sleep also start to hallucinate and are unable to concentrate effectively. The rest time associated with sleep allows for maintenance and repair of damaged body tissues. This is why it is important for people to get plenty of sleep when recovering from illness or injury. In children most growth occurs while they are asleep, so sleep is necessary for normal growth. While it is not clear in precise terms why sleep is necessary, it is known that animals deprived of sleep for long enough will die.

Changes in the CNS during sleep

Consciousness is generated in the brain stem in a structure referred to as the reticular activating system (RAS). Reduced activity of the RAS produces sleep, which is a state of partial unconsciousness. When the activity of the RAS is reduced the activity of the rest of the cerebral cortex is also reduced, as it is no longer being activated by the RAS.

Stages of sleep

NREM sleep is often described in four stages. Stage 1 is a transitional stage between waking and sleeping that normally only lasts for a few minutes when someone is falling to sleep. Stage 2 is the first stage of true sleep; it is a light sleep and fragmentary dreams may be experienced despite it being NREM. Stage 3 represents a moderately deep sleep and normally occurs about 20 minutes after falling asleep. In Stage 3 sleep, body temperature begins to fall, blood pressure decreases, and it is difficult to wake the person up. Stage 4 is deep sleep; the person responds only slowly if they are vigorously woken up.

After being in Stage 4 a person returns to Stage 3 then Stage 2 sleep, and after this there is a period of REM sleep. These sleep cycles tend to repeat about every 90 minutes and a person may dream for up to 2 hours per night.

Circadian rhythm

This is a pattern based on a 24-hour day cycle so it describes rhythms that occur on a daily basis, for example, waking and sleeping. Many physiological parameters have a circadian rhythm, e.g. body temperature drops at night. Urine production is reduced overnight and increased during the day. Metabolic rate is less during the night and several hormones have a circadian variation in serum levels.

Some thoughts

I hope you have now understood some of the physiological processes going on in the nervous system. If everything does not seem to make sense just now do not worry – much of the function of the brain is still a mystery to science. For example, I mentioned that the brain stem generates consciousness: we are aware of ourselves and our environment. The problem is how some nerve impulses and some neurochemicals can generate consciousness. Indeed, what is consciousness? We mentioned that sight is perceived in the occipital lobe. In a place where there is in fact no light at all we see all of the colours, textures and beauty of the world. When we do something we enjoy we feel pleasure but it seems this pleasure is just an increase in the activity of dopamine in the brain. Why should this give us pleasure?

Perhaps if all of these things cause us to reflect on the amazing nature and remaining mysteries of human physiology it is a good thing.

CHAPTER 3

The endocrine system

Introduction

A gland is a tissue or an organ that produces and secretes a chemical product. There are two forms of gland in the body, referred to as exocrine and endocrine. Before considering endocrine glands we will first think about exocrine glands.

Exocrine

'Exo-' means 'outside', so exocrine glands secrete products outside the internal environment. This means the products are secreted to the outside of the blood and tissue fluid, so are not systemically distributed (systemic means to do with the systems of the body).

Exocrine glands may be composed of one or many cells. Goblet cells provide a good example of the unicellular form of exocrine gland. These are cells that secrete mucus to lubricate internal surfaces. Goblet cells may be found in the epithelium of the respiratory, digestive, urinary and reproductive systems.

There are many different forms of multicellular exocrine glands but they all have secretory cells that secrete a product, and a duct that transports the product to a release site. For example a sweat gland produces sweat and a duct carries this product to the surface of the skin. Other examples of exocrine glands are mammary glands – milk, sebaceous glands – sebum, salivary glands – saliva, the pancreas – digestive enzymes, and the prostate gland – seminal fluid.

Diagram 3.1 A goblet cell in the lining of the gut. Mucus is secreted to protect and lubricate the lining of the gastrointestinal tract.

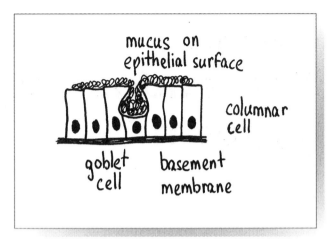

Diagram 3.2 Example of a coiled exocrine gland. Sweat is produced in the lower secretory portion then passes – through the duct – up to the surface.

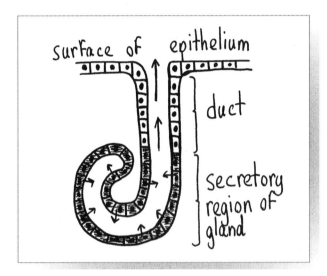

Endocrine

'Endo-' means 'inside'. Endocrine glands release their products directly into the blood and so into the internal environment. These glands have no ducts and in the past were called ductless glands for this reason. Endocrine products are released directly into the blood that is passing through the gland. This means that the endocrine products are rapidly systemically distributed.

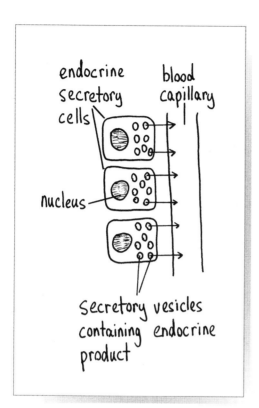

Diagram 3.3
Endocrine product is secreted directly into the blood. Arrows represent flow of endocrine product.

The products of endocrine glands are called hormones. A hormone is usually defined as a chemical messenger. After being produced in an endocrine gland a hormone circulates in the blood until it reaches a specific target tissue. The hormone then interacts with a receptor on the target tissue. The combination of the hormone and the receptor site then initiates a physiological response.

Signals and receptors

Because a hormone carries a chemical message it is sometimes referred to as a signal. A signal molecule has a particular shape and defined chemical properties. This means the signal will only bind to a specific receptor site. Receptor sites are made of protein and located on, or in, target cells. The hormone is analogous to a key, and the receptor to a lock. A specific key is required to open a particular lock. The cells that comprise the tissues of the body have many receptor sites on internal and external cell surfaces. However, only a signal with the correctly shaped 'key' can activate a specific receptor site. A target cell may have between 2 000 and 100 000 receptors for a particular hormone. Signal molecules may also be referred to as ligands.

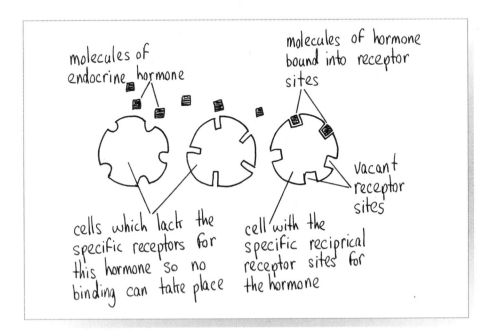

Diagram 3.4

The square-shaped signal molecule does not fit into the round or oblong receptor site. It can only fit into and bind with the reciprocally shaped receptor. Once the endocrine signal has bound to the receptor a physiological change will be initiated.

Endocrine glands

Hormones are produced by endocrine tissue, which is usually concentrated in specialized glands designed for this purpose (there are also a few hormones produced by endocrine tissue in organs which have another prime function).

Pituitary gland

The pituitary gland sits in the pituitary fossa, which is a small bony depression in the base of the skull. The gland is attached to the base of the brain underneath the hypothalamus. It is composed of two adjacent but separate lobes. The anterior lobe (to the front) is composed of glandular tissue. Anterior glandular tissue produces hormones and releases them directly into the blood.

The posterior lobe is made of neurological tissue; hormones released from this lobe are actually produced in cell bodies located in the hypothalamus. They travel down axons before release from the posterior lobe. Because posterior lobe hormones are produced in nerve cells the process is termed neurosecretion.

The scientifically correct name for the pituitary gland is the hypophysis. The anterior lobe is called the adenohypophysis because it is composed of glandular tissue ('adeno-' means 'to do with glandular tissue'). Because the posterior lobe is made of nervous tissue it is termed the neurohypophysis.

There are only two hormones secreted by the posterior lobe, oxytocin and antidiuretic hormone.

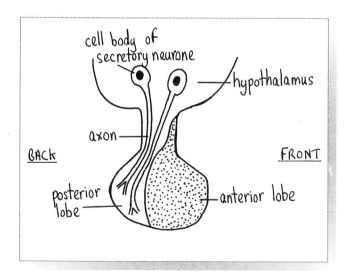

Diagram 3.5 Two lobes of the pituitary gland. Note the neurosecretory neurones arise in the hypothalamus and terminate in the posterior lobe.

Posterior pituitary hormones

Oxytocin

Release of this hormone may be stimulated by distension of the uterus in the later stages of pregnancy. Oxytocin then stimulates the contraction of the uterine muscles during labour. When a baby suckles at the nipple this also stimulates oxytocin release. In this case the hormone contracts the milk ducts to stimulate the release of milk from the nipple. In both cases oxytocin is working by stimulation of smooth muscle contractions.

Antidiuretic hormone (ADH)

Diuresis refers to the production of a large volume of urine. Diuretic drugs such as frusemide are given to increase urine volumes. An antidiuretic has the opposite effect: it acts against diuresis to reduce urine volumes. This means that the more ADH in the blood the less urine will be produced. In the absence of ADH the urine volumes will increase.

When the volume of water in the blood drops, this has the effect of increasing the concentration of the blood so increasing osmolarity; this is detected in the hypothalamus and causes ADH to be released. This hormone then travels to the kidneys in the blood. ADH acts on nephrons in the kidney to increase the volume of glomerular filtrate, which is reabsorbed back into the blood (see page 186). If the water from the glomerular filtrate is reabsorbed into the blood this means there is less left in the nephron to enter the urine. The result of this is that urine volume drops, so conserving water in the blood.

Conversely, if someone drinks large volumes of water, the blood will become too dilute, reducing blood osmolarity. This is detected in the hypothalamus and causes the pituitary gland to release less ADH. When there is less ADH in the blood, less water is reabsorbed from the glomerular filtrate in the nephron. This means more water is retained in the nephron so more water will pass on into the urine.

Alcohol inhibits the release of ADH; this means there is less antidiuretic effect, so urine volumes are large. This is why drinking alcohol causes dehydration (one of the causes of a hangover). Diabetes insipidus (nothing to do with diabetes mellitus) is a disease where there is a lack of ADH. This can result in a patient passing 20 litres of urine per day.

By regulating plasma levels of ADH the body is able to regulate the amount of water in the blood. This keeps the blood at the correct osmolarity. If the blood is too dilute the osmolarity will fall. In dehydration the osmolarity will tend to rise. This maintenance of equilibrium by ADH is an example of the principle of homeostasis ('homeo-' means 'same'). There are many parameters in the body that need to be maintained in the same state or at the same level, and homeostatic mechanisms exist to ensure this. We will see other examples of homeostasis later in this chapter and in subsequent chapters.

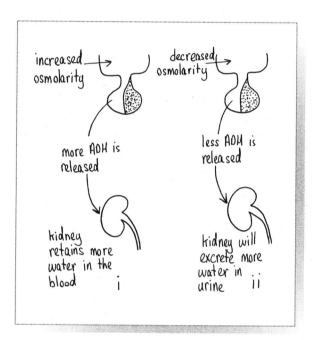

Diagram 3.6

(i) When blood osmolarity rises (i.e. there is less water in the blood) this is detected by the hypothalamus which causes more ADH to be released.

(ii) A reduction in blood osmolarity (this will happen when the blood is too dilute) will be detected by the hypothalamus, which reduces the amount of ADH released.

Anterior pituitary

The pituitary gland is often described as the master gland or 'the leader of the endocrine orchestra'; this is because the anterior lobe produces hormones that affect the activity of other endocrine glands. Many of these hormones are referred to by their initials.

Anterior pituitary hormones include thyroid-stimulating hormone (TSH); this is produced by a group of specialized anterior pituitary cells called thyrotrophs.

Adrenocorticotrophic hormone (ACTH) is produced by specialized cells called corticotrophs. Follicle-stimulating hormone (FSH)
and luteinizing hormone (LH) are produced by cells called
gonadotrophs. Prolactin is produced by lactotrophs and growth hormone (GH) by cells called somatotrophs.

Anterior pituitary hormones

Thyroid stimulating hormone (TSH)

Homeostasis refers to the maintenance of a constant internal environment; this is maintained in different ways in different parts of the
body. One group of parameters that needs to be finely regulated is
the levels of endocrine hormones in the blood. If these levels are
not kept relatively constant, the tissues of the body will be over- or
under-stimulated. One type of homeostatic mechanism is known as a
negative feedback system. An example of this is the control of the
amount of thyroid hormone (TH) in the blood. Low levels of thyroid
hormone in the blood are detected by specialized cells in the
hypothalamus. The hypothalamus responds to these low levels of TH
by releasing a substance called thyroid-stimulating hormone releasing
hormone (TSHRH). This TSHRH then stimulates the anterior lobe
of the pituitary gland to release another hormone, thyroid-
stimulating hormone (TSH). TSH then stimulates the thyroid gland
itself to produce thyroxin (thyroid hormone or TH). As the levels of
TH in the blood rise, the TH inhibits the release of further TSHRH
from the hypothalamus.

The underlying mechanism involved in this process is that
increased levels of thyroid hormone in the blood then inhibit the
release of its own initial releasing factor, i.e. the TSHRH. This is an
example of a negative feedback system. A negative feedback system is
when the end results of a process, e.g. TH, inhibit (have a negative
effect on) the release of the initial releasing factor for its own production – in this case TSHRH.

Adrenocorticotrophic hormone (ACTH)

This anterior pituitary hormone stimulates the release of hormones
from the adrenal cortex, both hydrocortisone and aldosterone. Levels

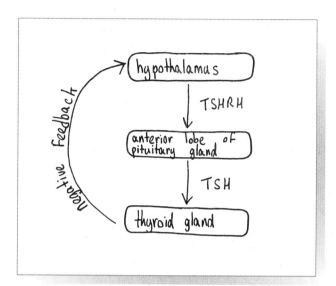

Diagram 3.7 The homeostatic control of TH levels in the blood via a negative feedback system. Rising levels of TH inhibit further release of TSHRH; falling levels of TH allow increased release of TSHRH.

of these hormones are detected by specialized cells in the hypothalamus in a similar way to the levels of thyroid hormone discussed above. The hypothalamus responds by secretion of the hormone that stimulates the release of ACTH – corticotrophin-releasing hormone (CRH). The CRH stimulates the release of ACTH from the anterior pituitary, and the ACTH then stimulates the release of the adrenal cortical hormones. The rise in the levels of adrenal cortical hormones inhibits the release of CRH from the hypothalamus. When this happens less ACTH is produced so less adrenal cortical hormones are released by the adrenal cortex. This is another example of the end product of a process inhibiting the release of its own initial releasing factor; in other words it is a negative feedback system. The end result of this mechanism is that plasma levels of adrenal cortical hormones are maintained at homeostatic levels.

Follicle-stimulating hormone (FSH)

FSH is an interesting hormone as it has different functions in men and women. In men, FSH stimulates the production of sperm in the testes by the process termed spermatogenesis. (The word 'genesis' refers to 'beginning' as in the first book of the Bible, so spermatogenesis is literally the beginning of sperm.)

In women, FSH has two functions. First, it stimulates the development of the ova each month in the ovaries. The structure containing the ova is called the follicle, from which FSH gets its name. An ovum is the egg cell, which can be fertilized by a sperm. Second, FSH stimulates the ovaries to release the female hormone, oestrogen.

Luteinizing hormone (LH)

This hormone again has a different function in the two sexes. In women, it stimulates the ovary to release an ovum, normally around day 14 of the menstrual cycle. LH also influences the secretion of oestrogen and progesterone. In men, LH stimulates the endocrine tissue in the testes to produce the male hormone, testosterone.

The release of FSH and LH are both regulated by the levels of a specific releasing hormone produced in the hypothalamus called gonadotrophin-releasing hormone (GnRH). Both FSH and LH are produced by the gonadotrophs of the anterior pituitary. This may be because they both act on the gonads.

Prolactin

Prolactin is also released as a result of stimulation by a hormone from the hypothalamus. In the case of prolactin, the releasing hormone is called prolactin-releasing hormone (PRH). PRH is released in response to the sucking action of an infant on the nipple. Prolactin acts on the breast to initiate and sustain the synthesis of milk; this process is called lactation. ('Lact-' means 'to do with milk'; for example lactose is the sugar found in milk.) In men, prolactin reduces blood levels of testosterone and at high levels may inhibit sperm production.

Growth hormone (GH)

GH is also sometimes called human growth hormone. It is the action of GH that causes children to grow. GH acts on body cells to stimulate the production of new proteins. In bone, this stimulation of protein synthesis leads to bone growth. If there is too much GH during development a giant will result; too little GH during childhood will lead to a dwarf. Most of the growth initiated by GH takes place at night; this is why it is very important that children get plenty of sleep.

So the anterior pituitary is a collection of different endocrine tissues, each composed of groups of specialized cells with specialized products, but all located in the same anatomical structure.

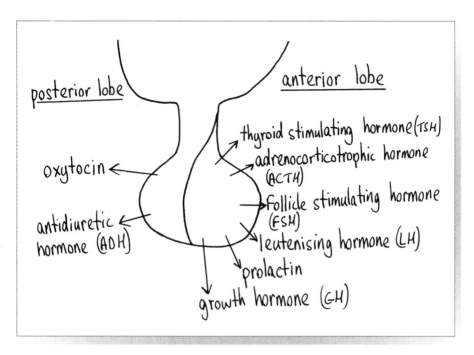

Diagram 3.8 Hormones
secreted from the two lobes
of the pituitary gland.

Hypothalamus

This part of the brain produces a range of hormones which act on the anterior pituitary and so must be considered to be endocrine. Most of these hormones stimulate the release of hormones from the pituitary gland, so they are often called releasing factors or releasing hormones. These include growth hormone releasing hormone (GHRH) and thyroid-stimulating hormone releasing hormone (TSHRH). These hormones pass through the pituitary gland before being diluted in the systemic blood circulation. They reach the pituitary in a network of veins called a portal system.

Thyroid gland

This endocrine gland is located in the neck just below the larynx. The gland consists of two lobes on either side of the thyroid cartilage and trachea. These two lobes are joined by a narrow section of thyroid tissue termed the thyroid isthmus. Two forms of secretory cells are contained in the thyroid gland. The most common ones are called follicular cells and these produce thyroid hormone. There are two forms of thyroid hormone: T3 contains three iodine atoms and T4 four iodine atoms in the molecule. Both of these thyroid hormones perform the same function but T3 is more potent.

From this, it is clear that iodine is essential for the formation of thyroid hormone. Iodine comes primarily from the sea, so people who do not have access to fish or sea salt may become deficient. In the UK this used to be common in Derbyshire because of its distance from the sea. When iodine is deficient the thyroid gland swells to try to extract more iodine from the blood. A swelling in the thyroid gland is called a goitre, and the traditional English name for this is Derbyshire neck. However, it is important to realize the thyroid gland may swell and produce toxic amounts of thyroid hormone; this pathological swelling is still referred to as a goitre.

The second form of secretory cells in the thyroid is the C cells, sometimes also called parafollicular cells. 'Para-' means 'beside', so these cells are beside the follicular cells. C cells secrete calcitonin.

Thyroid hormone

Secretion of the two forms of thyroid hormone is stimulated by TSH. Thyroid hormone acts on a wide range of body cells where it increases the metabolic rate. This means that thyroid-stimulated cells will use more glucose, fatty acids and oxygen to produce more energy. If a patient is over-producing thyroid hormone they will usually lose weight and feel hot. This is referred to as hyperthyroidism ('hyper-' means 'high'). Such patients lose weight because they use up their body's energy reserves. Whenever energy is used, heat is produced, explaining why the patients tend to feel hot. Conversely, if a patient has hypothyroidism ('hypo-' means 'low'), resulting in low levels of TH in the blood, they will tend to put on weight and feel cold, due to metabolic under-activity.

Thyroid hormone is also needed for the normal development of the brain. This is why if a person has low levels of thyroid hormone during the growing years, the brain does not develop normally, leading to mental retardation. In childhood, thyroid hormone is also needed for normal growth, so a child with low TH levels does not grow properly. This combination of stunted growth and mental retardation caused by childhood hypothyroidism is referred to as cretinism. This used to occur in the UK in areas where there was a deficiency of iodine in the diet. Hypothyroidism can now be readily treated with oral iodine or thyroxine.

Calcitonin

Secretion of calcitonin by the C cells of the thyroid is stimulated by increased levels of calcium in the blood. The calcitonin lowers plasma levels of calcium in two ways. First, it causes more calcium to be deposited in the bones. Second, calcitonin increases the excretion of calcium by the kidneys.

Parathyroid glands

There are four parathyroid glands located within the thyroid tissue but to the back of the thyroid gland itself. These produce parathyroid hormone (PTH).

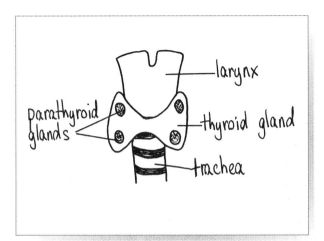

Diagram 3.9 Thyroid and parathyroids (the thyroid gland always reminds me of a bow tie).

Parathyroid hormone

This is produced by the parathyroid tissue in response to decreasing levels of calcium in the blood. Once released, parathyroid hormone increases plasma calcium levels in three ways. First, it increases the amount of calcium that is released from stores in the bone. Second, parathyroid hormone increases the amount of calcium that is reab-sorbed by the nephrons in the kidney, resulting in less calcium being lost in the urine. Third, it acts on the small intestine to increase the amount of calcium that is absorbed from food. If there is a deficiency of parathyroid hormone this will lead to reduced blood levels of calci-um. This hypocalcaemia causes muscle spasms, a condition called tetany. This is a rare complication of thyroid surgery and will occur if too much parathyroid tissue is accidentally removed. Tetany may be treated with calcium supplements.

It is this combined action of calcitonin lowering and parathyroid hormone raising blood calcium levels which maintains the mineral at homeostatic levels.

Thymus gland

This gland is located in the chest behind the sternum between the lungs. Several hormones are produced in the thymus such as thymosin and thymic factor.

Thymus hormone

Thymosis and thymic factor, secreted by the thymus gland, stimulate the maturation and activity of the T lymphocytes. These immune cells are discussed in detail in Chapter 13.

Pancreas

Endocrine tissue in the pancreas is located in the pancreatic islets (also called the islets of Langerhan). The pancreas is located in the upper area of the abdominal cavity behind the stomach. Most of the pancre-atic tissue produces exocrine digestive enzymes, which drain into the duodenum via the pancreatic duct. This means the pancreas has exocrine and endocrine functions. The islets form small 'islands' of tissue throughout the substance of the gland. Within each islet, or cluster of endocrine tissue, there are two main forms of cells called alpha and beta. The islets also contain cells called D and F.

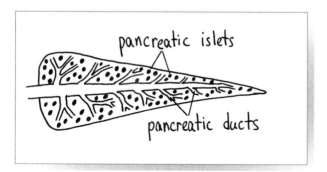

Diagram 3.10 Pancreas showing islet tissue. (The pancreas looks spotty – as if it has measles.)

Pancreatic islets

Another example of the endocrine system maintaining homeostasis is the physiology of blood glucose (sugar) regulation. If blood sugar levels drop too low, this condition is referred to as hypoglycaemia; if they rise too high this is referred to as hyperglycaemia. Both conditions are abnormal. The mechanisms of homeostasis maintain the concentration of glucose in the blood at a relatively constant normal physiological level.

When blood sugar levels are too high this is detected by the beta cells in the pancreatic islets (of Langerhan). The same beta cells respond by secreting the hormone insulin. Insulin goes into the blood and facilitates the conversion of soluble glucose to insoluble glycogen, which can then be stored in the liver and muscles. When glucose has been converted to glycogen and stored in this way it is no longer in the blood and blood sugar levels will therefore drop towards a normal homeostatic level.

In addition to this mechanism, insulin also facilitates the transfer of glucose across cell membranes, from the tissue fluids and blood into the cells of the body. In the absence of insulin, most cell membranes are impervious to the passage of glucose. The insulin molecule combines with receptor proteins in the cell membranes to open a channel or 'gate' through which glucose may pass. This means more glucose, under the influence of insulin, passes from the tissue fluids of the body into the cells. Once in the cells, glucose may be metabolized in the mitochondria to produce energy. Clearly, if the glucose is in the cells it

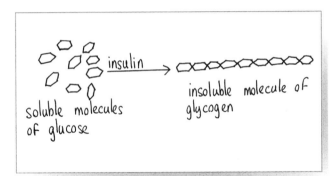

Diagram 3.11 Many molecules of soluble glucose are joined together under the influence of insulin to form a large glycogen molecule. Once formed, the large insoluble glycogen molecule may be stored in the liver or muscles.

is no longer in the blood, so again blood levels are lowered. The combination of these two mechanisms means the level of blood glucose drops back down towards a normal homeostatic level.

Conversely, when blood sugar levels are too low, this is detected in the alpha cells of the pancreatic islets. The same alpha cells respond by secreting a hormone called glucagon. Glucagon acts on stored glycogen to reconvert it back into glucose. This means insoluble glycogen, stored in the liver and muscles, is converted back into soluble

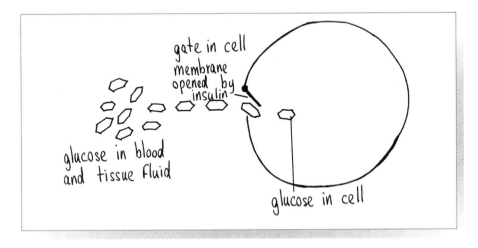

Diagram 3.12 Insulin gates the passage of glucose from tissue fluid into the cells.

glucose in the blood. The liberation of this soluble glucose raises blood sugar levels. In addition, low blood sugar levels will make the individual feel hungry, so he or she will eat if food is available. When the carbohydrate component of this food is absorbed it will also increase blood sugar levels.

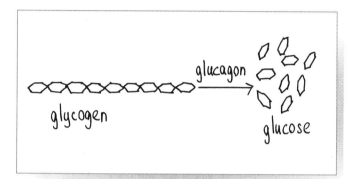

Diagram 3.13
The action of glucagon converting stored glycogen back into glucose.

In diabetes mellitus type 1 the beta cells die. This means the body can no longer produce insulin. The result of this is that blood sugar levels rise. However, the body cells are unable to receive the sugar that is in the blood and tissue fluids because there is no insulin to gate it across the cell membranes. Before insulin was isolated young people would die within several months of diagnosis.

Adrenal glands

The two adrenal glands are located one above each kidney. The outer layer of the adrenal gland is referred to as the cortex and the centre as the medulla. There are three layer or zones in the adrenal cortex. First, there is an outer layer that produces aldosterone. Underneath this, but still part of the cortex, is a layer that produces and secretes hydrocortisone (also called cortisol). The inner layer of the cortex produces sex hormones, mostly the male hormones called androgens. The medulla at the centre of the gland produces adrenaline and noradrenaline (i.e. epinephrine and norepinephrine).

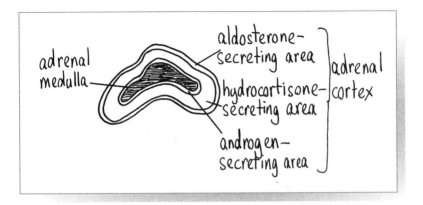

Diagram 3.14
The layers of the adrenal
glands, a central medulla
surrounded by three layers
of cortex.

Adrenal cortical hormones

Hydrocortisone is produced by the adrenal cortex. The function of
hydrocortisone is complex, but basically it increases the probability of
survival in difficult or dangerous situations. One function is to ensure
the body has enough available sources of energy to deal with times of
stress. This is why it increases the levels of nutrients in the blood, such
as amino acids, fatty acids and glucose. These nutrients are all required
to facilitate the metabolic reactions that produce energy, and will be
mobilized from body reserves if necessary. Glucose and fatty acids are
used by the body cells as fuels, while the amino acids may be synthesized into proteins which act as enzymes to facilitate metabolic
processes. In many survival situations the body may need to use large
amounts of energy over prolonged periods of time. This may be to
escape from predators or to seek out new sources of food.

Hydrocortisone also increases the probability of survival by inhibiting the inflammatory process. Inflammation is necessary for wound healing. However, inflammation also causes pain, which may inhibit essential
body movement and activity. Because hydrocortisone inhibits the inflammatory process it also inhibits pain. This means that movements essential to survival may carry on, such as fighting a predator or running away.

These mechanisms explain why levels of hydrocortisone are increased during periods of stress and anxiety. Hydrocortisone and other related steroid compounds may be given as drugs; in high doses they are very anti-inflammatory. This is sometimes a desirable therapeutic outcome.

The adrenal cortex also produces aldosterone. This has the effect of increasing the reabsorption of sodium from the renal nephrons so retaining more sodium in the blood. As sodium is an osmotic molecule it will tend to attract more water into the blood. This will increase overall blood volume and so will increase blood pressure. Again, in a survival situation, high plasma salt levels and consequent water levels will reduce the blood pressure lowering effects of haemorrhage. This means aldosterone will help to maintain blood pressure if blood is lost. If blood pressure is adequate, the perfusion of blood around vital organs such as the heart, lungs and brain will be maintained. Again this effect can increase the probability of surviving a difficult situation where blood has been lost.

Adrenal medullary hormones

Adrenaline and noradrenaline (also called epinephrine and norepinephrine) are both released from the adrenal medulla. Adrenaline works in a similar way to the sympathetic nervous system, to help the body to prepare rapidly for a flight or flight situation. Adrenaline will therefore increase the rate and force of cardiac contractions. It will dilate the bronchial passages to increase air entry to the alveoli. Blood supply to the skin and gut will be reduced by vasoconstriction to leave more blood for the skeletal muscles, heart and lungs. Adrenaline will also dilate the pupils of the eyes to increase light entry. Adrenaline even prepares the body for possible injury and blood loss by constricting peripheral blood vessels and by causing the blood to clot more quickly. Adrenaline and noradrenaline have similar effects, and the medulla secretes 80% adrenaline and 20% noradrenaline. The effects of adrenalin start a few seconds after the hormone is released; this means the body can be placed on an emergency footing as soon as danger is detected.

Kidneys

The prime function of the kidneys is to remove impurities from the blood and produce urine; however, the kidneys also have endocrine functions. Two hormones are produced by the kidney – erythropoi-etin and calcitriol. An enzyme called renin is also produced by the kidneys.

Erythropoietin

The kidneys are able to detect the amount of oxygen in the blood that is perfusing them. If levels of oxygen drop, the kidney responds by releasing erythropoietin. This hormone stimulates the process of erythropoiesis – the production of new erythrocytes or red blood cells. This cell-forming process takes place in the red bone marrow. If the number of red cells is increased this will increase the oxygen-carrying capacity of the blood, which should result in increasing levels of oxygen in the blood perfusing the kidneys. When the levels of oxygen in the renal blood supply are increased the kidney will secrete less erythropoietin. This regulation of the secretion of erythropoietin is therefore one of the mechanisms which controls the numbers of red cells and therefore influences the oxygen-carrying capacity of the blood.

In some cases of renal failure the kidney is no longer able to produce erythropoietin, resulting in anaemia. Some athletes have illegally used injections of synthesized erythropoietin to artificially increase the oxygen-carrying capacity of their blood to increase aerobic capacity. The erythropoietin mechanism also explains why people can adapt to high altitudes, where the partial pressure of oxygen is lower than at sea level. The danger of injecting synthesized erythropoietin or living at high altitude is that the increased numbers of red cells causes blood viscosity to increase. This in turn increases the probability of thrombosis formation (a thrombosis is a clot in a blood vessel and can result in death).

Calcitriol

The second hormone produced by the kidneys is calcitriol. This is in fact the active form of vitamin D. Inactive forms of vitamin D are generated in the skin when exposed to sunlight and absorbed from ingested food. However, the body is unable to use these forms until they have been activated in the kidney. Calcitriol is classified as a

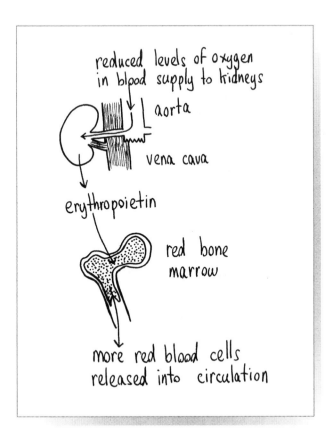

Diagram 3.15
Reduced levels of oxygen in renal arterial blood are detected and stimulate release of erythropoietin. Erythropoietin circulates in the blood to red bone marrow where it increases red cell production.

hormone because it is produced in the body from chemical precursors and is transported in the blood to target tissues. Loss of this ability to convert vitamin D to an active form explains why patients with chronic renal failure lose bone mass, as vitamin D is essential for normal bone metabolism. An enzyme called renin is also produced in the kidney and this is discussed in Chapter 9.

Gonads

Gonads is a collective term including both ovaries and testes. The ovaries are located in the female pelvis and the testes in the scrotal sack. Ovaries are responsible for the development and release of the ovum. They also produce two hormones, oestrogen and progesterone. The testes produce sperm and the principal male sex hormone called testosterone.

Ovarian hormones

The main hormones secreted by the ovaries are oestrogen and progesterone. Secretion of oestrogen is stimulated by the pituitary hormones FSH and LH. It is largely the increase in the blood levels of oestrogen that stimulates puberty in girls. Oestrogen causes development of the female reproductive organs as well as secondary sexual characteristics, such as breast development and body hair distribution. Oestrogen also promotes growth by stimulation of protein synthesis. Other functions of oestrogen are control of the menstrual cycle and development of the ovum and endometrium.

Like oestrogen, secretion of progesterone is stimulated by FSH and LH. Most progesterone is produced during the second half of the menstrual cycle. It is progesterone which maintains the development of the endometrium, so it is ready to receive and nourish an embryo, should one be formed during the menstrual cycle. Progesterone also stimulates growth of the mammary glands (in the breasts) ready for milk secretion.

During pregnancy, oestrogen and progesterone are also produced by the placenta, the structure connecting the mother and the baby. The role of the placenta is to allow the diffusion of oxygen and nutrients from mother to baby and the passage of carbon dioxide and waste products of metabolism from baby to mother. Oestrogen and progesterone secreted by the placenta maintain the lining of the uterus and prepare the breasts to secrete milk. During pregnancy, high levels of oestrogen and progesterone prevent further pregnancies by inhibiting ovulation. Combined oral contraceptive pills work by artificially increasing blood levels of oestrogen and progesterone to inhibit ovulation and therefore prevent conception.

Testicular hormones

The testes are located in the scrotal sack and produce testosterone. Secretion of testosterone is stimulated by LH. Increasing levels of testosterone stimulate puberty in boys. The hormone causes development of external genitalia and stimulates sperm production. By promoting protein synthesis, testosterone stimulates growth of the body and muscles. It also leads to male secondary sexual characteristics such as deepening of the voice and the growth of facial hair.

CHAPTER 4

The cardiovascular system

The heart

Basic structure

The heart is a hollow organ located in the centre and extending to the left of the thoracic cavity. With the sternum and ribs to the front and the thoracic spinal column behind, the heart is well protected from physical trauma. Within the heart there are four chambers. The two upper chambers are termed atria and the lower chambers ventricles. These chambers are named according to the side of the heart they are on, so they are the right and left atria and the right and left ventricles.

The atria and ventricles are separated by valves collectively referred to as atrioventricular valves. On the right side, the atrioventricular valve is called the tricuspid valve. This is because it is made up of three separate cusps. The bicuspid valve is between the left atrium and ventricle and is composed of two cusps. Often the bicuspid valve is alternatively referred to as the mitral valve.

Diagram 4.1

(i) View of the closed tricuspid valve from above.

(ii) View of the closed bicuspid (mitral) valve from above.

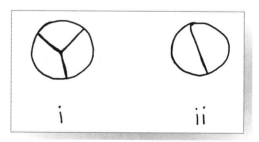

Valves are essential to control the direction of blood flow through the heart. A valve will only allow the blood to flow in one direction. Heart valves are attached to the ventricular wall by strong tendons called chordae tendineae, or tendonous cords. These prevent the valves opening upwards, the wrong way. The chordae tendineae are themselves connected to the wall of the heart via specialized muscle bundles called papillary muscles.

The heart is a pump. Atria act as receiving chambers for the venous blood which is returning to the heart. Ventricles are pumping chambers that pump blood into the arteries. The left ventricle pumps blood into the main artery supplying blood to the body; this large vessel is referred to as the aorta. The right ventricle pumps blood into the main artery supplying blood to the lungs, called the pulmonary artery ('pulmonary' always means 'to do with the lungs'). Shortly after leaving the right ventricle, the pulmonary artery divides into two main branches, one to each lung. Between the left ventricle and the aorta is a valve called the aortic valve (in older texts you may see this referred

Diagram 4.2 The basic structures of the heart.

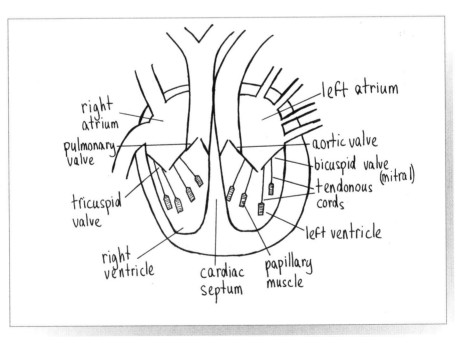

to as the aortic semilunar valve). Between the right ventricle and the pulmonary artery is the pulmonary valve (also sometimes referred to as the pulmonary semilunar valve).

The left and right sides of the heart are separated by the cardiac septum. This means that blood from the right side cannot mix with blood from the left side, and vice versa.

Blood flow through the heart and around the body

The heart is essentially two pumps. The left side pumps blood to the body and the right side to the lungs. Blood is pumped to the lungs to be oxygenated and to excrete ('excrete' just means 'to get rid of') carbon dioxide. Haemoglobin in red blood cells absorbs oxygen from the lungs, and this oxygenated blood will then return to the left side of the heart via the pulmonary veins. The four pulmonary veins, two from each lung, drain blood into the left atrium. From the left atrium, blood passes through the bicuspid valve into the left ventricle. The atrium contracts to aid the passage of blood into the ventricle. After atrial contraction, the ventricle contracts; this has the effect of increasing the pressure of the blood in the ventricle, which causes the closure of the bicuspid valve. This closure prevents the blood being pumped from the ventricle back into the atrium. The increase in the blood pressure in the ventricle caused by its contraction also causes the opening of the aortic valve, which allows blood to be pumped into the aorta. After ventricular contraction, back-flow from the aorta into the left ventricle is prevented by the closure of the aortic valve. From the aorta blood then passes, via the arterial system, to all the tissues of the body.

As the blood circulates around the body it gives up oxygen to the tissues, and veins then collect the blood and return it to the heart. The systemic veins drain blood into two large central veins called the superior and inferior vena cava. These two veins drain the top and bottom halves of the body respectively. They both drain directly into the right atrium. From the right atrium the blood passes through the tricuspid valve into the right ventricle, again aided by atrial contraction. When the right ventricle contracts this causes the closure of the tricuspid valve and the opening of the pulmonary valve. This means blood will be pumped into the pulmonary artery, and on to the lungs. Back-flow from the pulmonary artery into the right ventricle is prevented by the pulmonary valve.

The order of the circulation of the blood can be summarized as follows: left ventricle – aortic valve – aorta – body – vena cava – right atrium – tricuspid valve – right ventricle – pulmonary valve – lungs – pulmonary vein – left atrium – bicuspid valve – left ventricle.

Both sides of the heart contract together, simultaneously pumping blood to lungs and body.

Arterial blood in the systemic circulation is bright red because it is rich in oxyhaemoglobin, a bright red pigment. This is because the blood has passed through the lungs and is fully oxygenated. However, in the pulmonary arteries, the blood is on the way to the lungs to be oxygenated, after giving up its oxygen to the tissues of the body. This is why blood in the pulmonary arteries is dark red and deoxygenated. Blood in the systemic veins is dark red, compared to blood in the pulmonary veins, which is bright red and fully oxygenated.

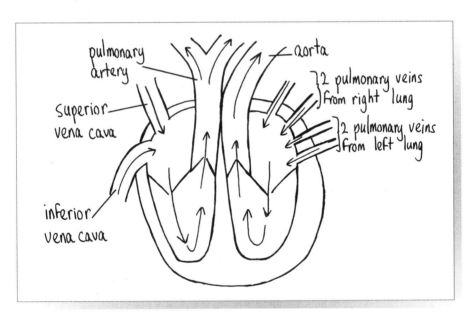

Diagram 4.3 The major blood vessels associated with the heart, arrows indicate direction of blood flow.

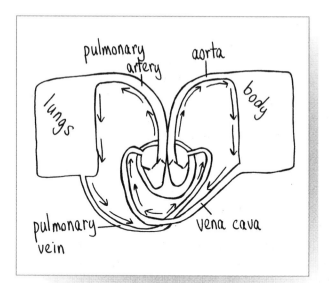

Diagram 4.4
This simplified diagram shows the flow of the blood through the heart and around the body and the lungs. (You may find it helpful to colour these diagrams in. The tradition is red for oxygenated blood and blue for deoxygenated.)

Heart valves are passive structures that open and close in response to pressure changes in the four heart chambers. This principle of pressure changes within the heart opening and closing valves is applied when carrying out external cardiac massage. This compresses the heart between the thoracic vertebral column and the sternum. As the pressure in the heart increases, blood will open the valves and be forced through. As valves only allow the blood to flow one way, the circulation can only occur in a physiological direction. Cardiac massage will generate a cardiac output that may be detected as a central pulse. This will perfuse the vital organs of the body such as the lungs, brain, kidneys and the heart itself. This can be maintained until a normal cardiac rhythm is restored.

The muscle mass of the left ventricle is greater than that of the right. This is because the pressure required to perfuse the body is greater than that needed to pump blood to the lungs. A typical pressure in the systemic circulation is 120/80 mmHg whereas in the pulmonary circulation it is 25/8 mmHg. The first figure represents the blood pressure in the arteries when the heart is contracting and is referred to as the systolic pressure. The second figure is the pressure in the arteries when there is no active cardiac contraction, in between beats. This second pressure reflects the elasticity of the arterial system and is termed the diastolic pressure.

Heart sounds

Both atrioventricular valves close at the same time, making a sound referred to as a 'lub'. The closure of the two arterial semilunar valves makes a 'dub'. These are termed the first and second heart sounds, so the normal heart should make a 'lub dub, lub dub, lub dub'. Heart sounds can easily be heard with a stethoscope. Additional sounds may be abnormal and are often caused by disturbances in the smooth flow of blood. An abnormal heart sound referred to as a 'whoosh' is often heard in septal defects where there is a communication between the right and left sides of the heart (a 'hole in the heart'). The resultant mixing of oxygenated and deoxygenated blood reduces the efficiency of the circulatory system. In this case, some oxygenated blood is returned to the lungs and some deoxygenated blood is pumped into the systemic circulation. Such conditions are usually congenital and require surgical correction.

Three layers

The inner layer of the heart is called the endocardium and is composed of smooth squamous epithelium. This allows the smooth uninterrupt-ed flow of blood through the heart. Endocardium also covers the heart valves. The importance of this epithelium is highlighted by the effect of its becoming infected, a condition termed endocarditis. Usually caused by a streptococcus, this condition causes inflammation fol-lowed by deposits of the blood-clotting protein, fibrin, which cause the build up of 'vegetation'. If this material is dislodged it will enter the circulatory system as emboli which can lodge in the small arterial supply of any part of the body.

The energy for the pumping action is generated by the heart mus-cle, which is called the myocardium. This cardiac form of muscle is only found in the heart; it is striped or striated in nature but unlike skeletal muscle it is involuntary. The myocardium is the middle layer of the heart wall. As the myocardium must contract approximately 72 times per minute it uses a lot of nutrients and oxygen.

The other layer of the heart is termed the pericardium and is com-posed of two layers. The inner layer is composed of serous membrane, which is adherent to the outside of the myocardium and is referred to as the visceral pericardium or epicardium. The outer layer is composed of tough fibrous tissue, which is itself lined internally with another layer of serous membrane. A serous membrane is a membrane that secretes serous lubrication fluid, in this case to allow the heart to move within the fibrous pericardial sack without any friction between layers. This allows the heart to expand and contract during a normal cardiac cycle. The fibrous layer is protective and prevents the heart over-expanding. If fluid or blood collects under the fibrous pericardium the pressure can squash the heart and may cause death. This condition is termed cardiac tamponade.

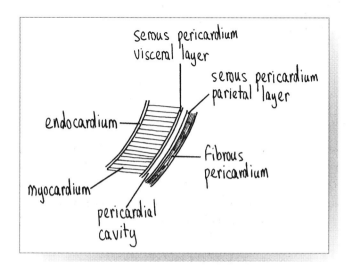

Diagram 4.5 The three layers which compose the wall of the heart.

Coronary arteries

The first two arteries to leave the aorta are the right and left coronary arteries; these supply the arterial system of the myocardium. Coronary arteries supply the myocardium with blood and therefore oxygen and nutrients. Disease of these arteries is termed coronary artery disease and is the single most common cause of death in the western world. This disease occurs when the lumen of the arteries is clogged up with a cholesterol-based material called atheroma. Because the atheroma blocks off part of the lumen, less blood is able to get through to the myocardium: this reduction in blood supply is called ischaemia. In addition, the atheroma increases the probability that a blood clot may form in the lumen of the artery: this pathological condition is referred to as thrombosis. Clinically, these consequences of atheroma may cause angina and myocardial infarction.

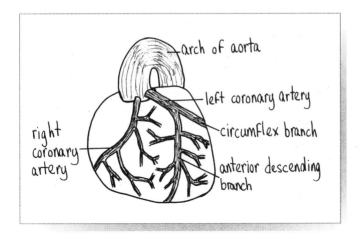

Diagram 4.6
The main coronary
arteries.

The cardiac cycle

A cardiac cycle is one complete contraction and relaxation of the heart, and comprises the events that take place during one heartbeat. The heart contracts at a regular rate from about 8 weeks after conception until the death of the individual. Heart rate varies with the age of the person from about 140 per minute at birth to around 110 at age 2, 80 at age 10 and around 70 in adults.

The internal electrical conducting system

The cardiac cycle is controlled by specialized conducting tissue in the heart. Inside the right atrium is an area of specialized cardiac muscle tissue termed the sinoatrial (SA) node (because this controls the pace of the heart it is sometimes called the pacemaker). This area generates the initial electrical impulse to stimulate myocardial contraction. From the SA node an impulse spreads to both atria stimulating their contraction. The impulse travels across the atria via specialized conduction pathways termed the internodal tracts – because they are between the SA node and the atrioventricular (AV) node.

The AV node collects the impulse from the atria and passes it on to the bundle of His (or atrioventricular bundle) in the cardiac septum. The AV node is the only way the impulse can spread from the atria to the ventricles, since the rest of the tissue in the plane of the valves is electrically insulating. In the cardiac septum the bundle of

His divides into two, forming the right and left bundle branches, which carry the impulse to the right and left ventricles. The result of this arrangement is that the impulse is carried rapidly down through the cardiac septum. Finally the impulse innervates the ventricular myocardial muscle via the small Purkinje fibres (or conduction myo-fibres). This means that ventricular contraction will start from the bottom and work up, pushing the blood upwards, towards the arterial valves. It is this internal conducting system that is responsible for the initiation and the phases of the cardiac cycle.

Unlike other muscles, the heart generates the electrical impulses that lead to muscle contraction internally. This is why a donated heart can carry on contracting after a heart transplant operation. However, outside factors will influence the heart rate and strength of contraction. Adrenaline will increase heart rate, as will stimulation by the sympathetic nervous system. Parasympathetic stimulation will slow heart rate and so reduce cardiac output.

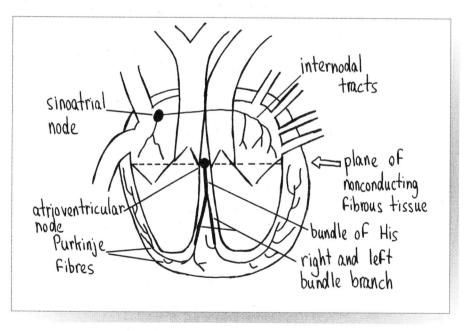

Diagram 4.7 The components of the cardiac internal conducting system. An electrical impulse can only pass through the non-conducting fibrous tissue of the valvular plane via the AV node.

The PQRST

When the myocardium is stimulated by the Purkinje fibres, the myocardial cells will depolarize. (The physiology of polarization was discussed in Chapter 2.) It is the depolarization of the myocardial cells that initiates contraction. This collective electrical activity may be detected with electrodes on the surface of the body. In health the depolarization of the muscle will occur essentially at the same time as contraction of the myocardium. This is the principle of the electrocardiogram (ECG). When this is recorded three characteristic electrical phases can be clearly seen.

First, there is a P wave. This is the electrical activity, as detected on the surface of the body, as a result of the depolarization of the atrial myocardium.

Second, there is the larger QRS complex caused by the depolarization of the larger muscle mass of the ventricular myocardium; this complex is associated with ventricular contraction. Third, there is a T wave. This is not associated with any muscular contraction but arises

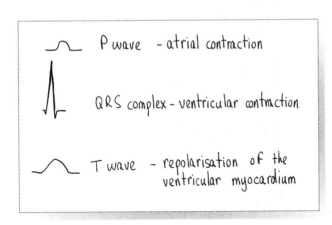

Diagram 4.8
The components of the cardiac cycle and the events represented by the electrical activity.

Diagram 4.9
A normal ECG recorded from one of my students.

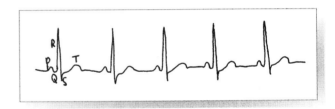

as the ventricular muscle repolarizes to an electrically resting state. Finally, there is a short gap before the next atrial contraction.

A normal cardiac cycle must have a PQRST phase in that order. In health the occurrence of these phases of the cycle is fairly regular and the rate is usually between 60 and 100 per minute. So a normal rhythm has a PQRST, in the correct order, which is regular, with a rate between 60 to 100 cycles per minute. This normal rhythm is called a sinus rhythm because the cardiac rhythm is controlled by the sinoatrial atrial node.

If the phases of the cardiac cycle occur regularly, and in the correct order, at a rate of less than 60 times per minute, the rhythm is termed sinus bradycardia. This is normal in people who are physically fit. If the rate is over 100, with a regular PQRST in the right order, this is termed a sinus tachycardia. A sinus tachycardia is of course normal during exercise.

The terms P, Q, R, S and T do not stand for anything and have no intrinsic significance whatsoever. They are arbitrary names given to specified phases.

Effects of exercise

Exercise increases heart rate, which is the number of times the heart beats per minute. It also increases stroke volume, which is the amount of blood pumped out per cardiac contraction. These two factors combine to increase cardiac output, which is defined as the volume of blood pumped out from the left ventricle per minute. To be precise, cardiac output equals heart rate × stroke volume. At rest a normal stroke volume will be around 70 ml; if the heart rate is 72 beats per minute this would give a cardiac output of 70 × 72, which equals a cardiac output of 5040 ml. During vigorous exercise cardiac output may rise as high as 35 litres per minute.

Regular exercise is very good for people. It lowers harmful fats in the blood and helps keep blood pressure down. It also makes the heart muscle stronger and helps to keep the coronary arteries patent. Exercise also tones and strengthens many other muscles in the body. If people are immobilized and unable to exercise they may suffer from numerous complications such as blood clots in the veins of the legs and lungs, pressure sores, depression, constipation, pneumonia and atrophy of bones and muscles. This is why everyone should try to exercise for at least half an hour every day.

The blood vessels

The main types of blood vessels are arteries, arterioles, capillaries, venules and veins.

Arteries

An artery is any vessel that carries blood away from the heart. Essentially, arteries are tubes that supply an area of tissue with blood. This is vital; if an area is deprived of a regular blood supply the tissues will die because all of the oxygen and nutrients the cells require are transported to them in the blood. Larger arteries divide into smaller arteries so the whole of the body can be perfused with blood.

Arteries have fairly thick walls because the blood they carry is at relatively high pressure. If an artery is cut, the blood initially comes out in spurts. Fortunately, most arteries are deep in the body for protection. Because the arteries carry blood directly from the heart, a pulse can be felt every time the heart contracts.

Arterial walls consist of three layers. First, the tunica externa (also called tunica adventitia) is the external or outer layer; this is composed mostly of connective tissues, containing collagen and elastic fibres. Second, the tunica media is the middle layer; this contains elastic fibres and smooth muscle. The third inner layer is called the tunica interna; this is a layer of smooth squamous endothelium to allow smooth flow of blood ('tunica' means 'coat'). The hole in the middle of any vessel is referred to as the lumen.

All of the systemic arteries branch from the aorta. The carotid arteries can be felt in the neck and supply the head with blood. Blood pressure is usually recorded from the brachial artery supplying the arm. The femoral pulse can be felt in the groin. Behind the knee, the pulse of the popliteal artery can be felt. The most common pulse felt by nurses is the radial, where the radial artery passes over the radius. However, in cardiovascular emergency situations it may not be possible to feel the radial pulse, so we should always assess a central pulse, usually the carotid or femoral. Other main arteries include the intercostal arteries to the intercostal muscles, the hepatic artery to the liver, and the renal arteries to the kidneys.

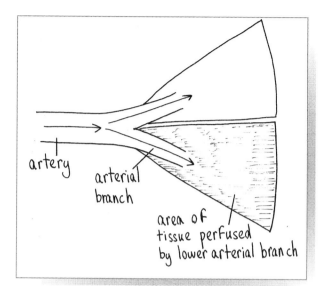

Diagram 4.10 An artery supplying an area of tissue with blood. (Often an arterial branch will supply a wedge-shaped area of tissue.)

Diagram 4.11
Cross-section of an artery to show the three layers and lumen.

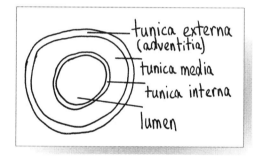

Arterioles

Small arteries divide into even smaller arterial vessels called arterioles. These vessels are almost microscopic and carry blood into the microscopic capillaries. Arterioles contain circular smooth muscle fibres in their walls that allow them to dilate and constrict. This vasodilation and vasoconstriction allows for the regulation of the flow of blood through a tissue ('vaso-' means 'to do with blood vessels'). For example, after a heavy meal the arterioles to the gut will dilate (i.e. widen); this will increase the volumes of blood perfusing capillaries of the gut wall. During exercise the arterioles to the skeletal muscles will dilate to increase their blood supply. When someone is cold the arterioles supplying the skin capillary beds will vasoconstrict to reduce the amount of warm blood near the surface of the skin.

Arterioles are important in the regulation of blood pressure. Widespread constriction of the arterioles will narrow the total lumen of the arterial system; this in turn will increase resistance to blood flow. The resistance to blood flow offered by the arterioles is termed peripheral resistance. Conversely, if the arterioles are dilated, there will be less resistance to blood flow and peripheral resistance will be reduced.

If peripheral resistance is increased blood pressure will also be increased. Conversely, if peripheral resistance is lowered due to vasodilation, blood pressure will be lowered. The other factor influencing blood pressure is the amount of blood pumped out by the heart. So blood pressure may be precisely defined as cardiac output multiplied by peripheral resistance.

The relative tone of the arterioles is regulated by a specialized area in the medulla oblongata (part of the brain stem) called the vasomotor centre. This regulation of blood pressure is essential for life. If blood pressure is too low, tissues will not be adequately perfused. For example, if the brain is acutely hypoperfused a person will faint. However, if blood pressure is too high this will damage the walls of the arteries leading to possible haemorrhage; hypertension will also contribute to atheroma formation.

Capillaries

Capillaries are the smallest blood vessels and are microscopic; they receive blood from the arterioles. Capillaries are the only part of the circulatory system where there is exchange of materials from the blood to the tissues or from the tissues to the blood – all other vessel walls are too thick to allow diffusion. Capillaries, however, are able to facilitate this exchange because they are only one squamous cell thick, which means the diffusional distance between the blood and the tissue cells is very small, allowing relatively free diffusion.

Living tissue contains millions of capillaries arranged in beds. A capillary bed refers to a system of capillaries perfusing a particular area of tissue. For example, fingernail beds are pink because of the colour of the blood passing through a capillary bed. If you press on your fingernails, the beds turn white. This is because the pressure of the nail from above has squeezed the blood out of the capillary bed so the pink colour is lost. Overall, the capillaries form a massive surface area between the blood and the tissues: it has been suggested that the total area of capillary wall in an adult is 6 000 square metres.

The exchange of material between the blood and tissue fluid is aided by small gaps which are present between some of the capillary cells. These gaps are called capillary pores.

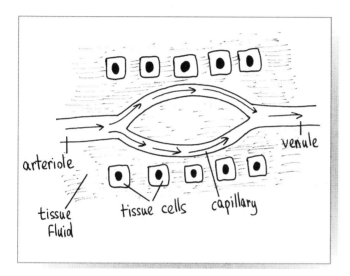

Diagram 4.12

An arteriole divides into a group of capillaries which perfuse some tissue cells.

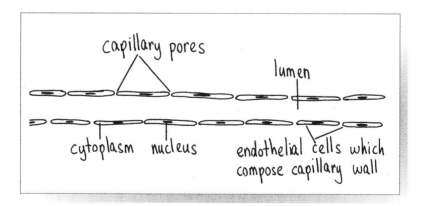

Diagram 4.13

A magnified view of a capillary wall made up of individual endothelial cells.

Tissue fluid

As can be seen from Diagram 4.12, the cells of a tissue are bathed in tissue fluid. This is essential to keep the cells moist and to prevent them drying out. In addition, tissue fluid is an essential medium for diffusion between the blood and capillaries. Substances diffuse from the blood, through the tissue fluid before reaching and diffusing into cells. The same is true for substances the cells excrete. These waste products must diffuse into the tissue fluid before they can diffuse through the capillary wall into the blood.

It is the capillaries that are responsible for the formation of the tissue fluid. At the arteriole end of the capillary, because the blood has recently left the arterial system, the blood pressure is still relatively high. Because the pressure in the capillary is greater than in the tissue fluid, water molecules that are small enough to fit through the capillary pores are forced out from the capillary blood into the tissue spaces. Larger components of the blood such as cells and plasma proteins, which are big molecules, remain in the capillaries. Once formed, tissue fluid bathes and flows over the individual tissue cells.

At the venous end of the capillary blood pressure is lower because the blood is nearing the lower pressure venous system. Because blood plasma contains large protein molecules, the plasma generates an

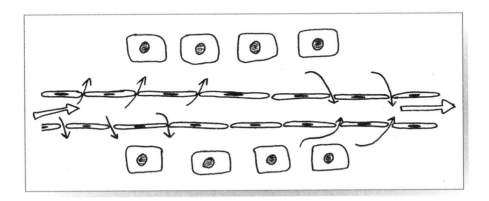

Diagram 4.14 Formation and reabsorption of tissue fluid, water is exuded from the arterial end of the capillary, washes over the tissue cells and is reabsorbed at the venous end of the capillary. Dark arrows represent tissue fluid movement, white arrows indicate direction of blood flow.

osmotic pressure that tends to suck in water. At the venous end of the capillary, the osmotic pressure is greater than the blood pressure that is trying to force water molecules out of the capillary. The net effect of this is that water molecules are osmotically drawn back into the blood at the venous end of the capillary. The overall result of this process of tissue fluid formation and reabsorption is that there is a flow of fresh tissue fluid over the tissue cells, from the arteriole to the venous end of the capillary. This flow helps keep tissue cells nourished and oxygenated as well as removing toxic waste products.

When the levels of protein in the blood are very low, as in severe malnutrition, the plasma is no longer able to generate the osmotic pressure required to reabsorbed tissue fluid. This is why people with severe protein deficiencies develop oedema (the retention of fluid in the tissues).

Gaseous exchange

Capillaries are the site of gaseous exchange between the blood and tissues. All living tissues need a constant supply of oxygen to allow mitochondria to produce the energy essential for life. In the systemic circulation, arterial blood arrives from the arterioles containing high concentrations of oxygen. Because the tissues have been using up oxygen, the concentration in cells is relatively low. This means there will be a diffusion gradient between the high level of oxygen in the blood and lower levels in the tissues. The result of this is that oxygen will diffuse from the blood into the tissue cells.

The same principle of differential concentrations of dissolved gas also determines the movement of carbon dioxide. Ongoing metabolism in the cells produces carbon dioxide, the concentration of which will tend to rise. Arterial blood arrives from the arterioles containing very low concentrations of carbon dioxide. This means there is a concentration gradient from the cells to the blood, resulting in the diffusion of carbon dioxide from tissues into the blood. By these mechanisms the cells maintain oxygenation and dispose of waste carbon dioxide.

In addition to gaseous exchange, nutrients that cells require diffuse from the blood to the cells, through the capillary walls and tissue fluids. Nutrients include amino acids, fatty acids, glucose, minerals and vitamins. As well as producing waste carbon dioxide, cells produce other chemical wastes as a result of their metabolic processes: these

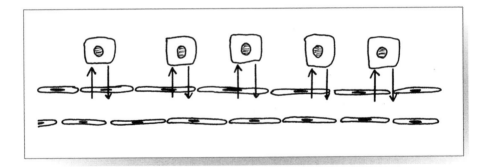

Diagram 4.15 Gaseous exchange between blood and tissues. Oxygen diffuses from capillary blood to tissue cells and carbon dioxide from cells to blood.

include waste nitrogen-containing toxic molecules such as ammonia. If these were allowed to accumulate in the tissues they would eventually poison the cells.

Veins

A vein may be defined as any vessel that carries blood towards the heart. Veins have the same basic three-layered structure as arteries, with a central lumen, tunica interna, media and externa. Because the pressure of blood in the veins is lower than in arteries, the walls are thinner.

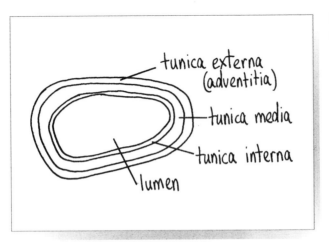

Diagram 4.16
A cross-section of a vein.

Unlike arteries, veins have valves within their lumen to prevent back flow of blood. If veins are damaged, dark red blood oozes out, as opposed to the spurting of bright red blood from a freshly cut artery. Systemic veins carry deoxygenated blood and the pulmonary veins carry oxygenated blood.

Mechanisms of venous return

Blood flows along the arteries because of the pumping effect of the heart generating a blood pressure. However, once blood has passed through the capillaries, virtually all of this pressure is lost. In veins above the heart, blood can return to the right atrium under the influence of gravity; however, for veins below the level of the heart, extra mechanisms of venous return are needed. The mechanisms of venous return are contraction of adjacent muscles, contraction of adjacent arteries and negative and positive pressures set up in the thorax and abdomen during respiration. All of these mechanisms rely on the action of valves in the veins. These prevent back-flow of blood from the centre to the periphery. Any blood trying to flow backwards will have the effect of closing off the valve immediately below. The importance of venous valves is clearly illustrated in varicose veins where there is failure of the valves and pooling of blood dilates the veins.

The most dramatic mechanism of venous return is contraction of adjacent muscles. This works especially well for deep veins that run

Diagram 4.17

A series of valves in peripheral veins. Blood flowing upwards (towards the heart) will automatically open the valves whereas blood flowing backwards will close them. Arrows indicate the direction of blood flow.

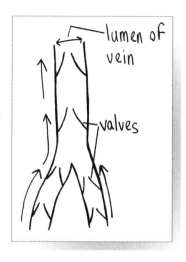

through muscles. When a muscle contracts, veins within the muscle are squeezed; this has the effect of raising the pressure in the lumen of the vein. This will close the valves below the area of increased pressure and force blood upwards, towards the centre. This mechanism works so efficiently in the calf muscles it is referred to as the calf muscle pump. This is why it is important for patients on bed rest to keep their ankles moving – to activate the calf pump so preventing pooling of blood in the legs.

Veins, arteries and nerves often run together in the body, usually in areas where they are protected from outside trauma. For example, the main vein and artery in the upper leg lie behind the quadriceps muscle and femur; this means they are protected from most blows or

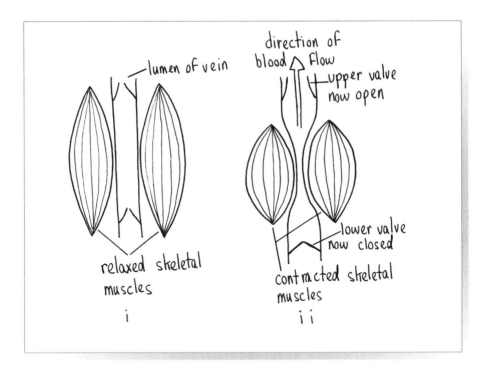

Diagram 4.18
The action of the calf muscle pump; muscle contraction shortens the muscle which squeezes the vein running through.
(i) A deep vein in a muscle that is relaxed.
(ii) A deep vein in a muscle that is contracting.

traumas coming from outside. This is why the upper outer aspect of the thigh is a safe site for intramuscular injections: the needle is unlikely to hit a nerve, artery or vein. Because arteries pulsate, they press on adjacent veins and so slightly squeeze them; this will increase the pressure of the blood in the lumen of the vein and so aid venous return. This is a less dramatic mechanism than skeletal muscle contraction but it is constant.

During inspiration the diaphragm moves down. As the diaphragm is between the thorax and the abdomen, downward movement compresses the abdominal contents. Because the inferior vena cava runs through the abdomen, this will be slightly compressed during inspiration. This pressure on the vena cava will increase the pressure of the blood it contains, closing the valves beneath, while pumping blood back into the thoracic cavity. Also during inspiration, because the diaphragm moves down, and the ribs move up and out, the pressure in the thorax is reduced. This reduction in pressure sucks blood into the thoracic vena cava from the abdominal vena cava.

During expiration, because the diaphragm moves up, the pressure in the abdomen is lowered. This allows blood from the leg veins to pass up, into the abdominal vena cava. The pressure in the thorax increases during expiration, because the diaphragm moves up and the ribs move down and in. This increase in thoracic pressure means the pressure in the thoracic vena cava will also increase. This has the effect of squeezing blood from the thoracic vena cava back into the right atrium.

Clinical applications

The mechanisms of venous return described above are one reason why patients on bed rest should be advised to take regular deep breaths, as well as keeping their ankles moving. If venous return is too sluggish there is the possibility of a blood clot forming in the deep veins, a condition referred to as deep venous thrombosis. This is very painful, but the real danger is that part of the blood clot will break off and form an embolus. This will travel with the venous blood back through the right side of the heart and will become jammed in a branch of the pulmonary artery. This condition is referred to as pulmonary embolism and is life-threatening.

As well as the deep veins, in the limbs there are also superficial veins, just under the skin. It is safe to put a tourniquet on the upper arm for a couple of minutes. This will restrict venous return, and so the veins will fill up with blood. In this state they are easy to feel. This palpation of veins is a vital skill, if nurses want to gain venous access for taking blood samples or inserting venous cannulas.

Some veins you may come across in clinical practice include the jugular in the neck and the subclavian under the clavicle. Venous cannulas are often sited in the cephalic vein, over the lateral surface of the radius. The femoral veins drain blood from the legs and the renal veins carry blood from the kidneys directly to the inferior vena cava.

Portal veins

A portal vein is one that does not drain into a larger vein but ends in capillaries. There is a portal system between the hypothalamus and the anterior pituitary to carry hypothalamic releasing hormones. As blood is passing directly from one area to another it is not diluted in the entire blood volume. This means smaller volumes of hormone may be used to generate the desired physiological effect, which increases the efficiency of the process. The other main example of a portal system is the hepatic portal vein. Blood draining from the stomach, small and large intestine is collected together into this single vessel. The result of this is that all of the blood drained from the gut passes directly into the liver; only once this blood has circulated through the liver does it

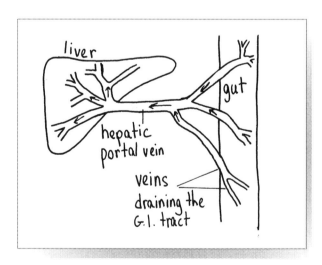

Diagram 4.19
Blood draining from the gastrointestinal tract carries absorbed nutrients and bacterial toxins directly to the liver for biochemical processing. Arrows indicate direction of blood flow.

enter the inferior vena cava via the hepatic vein. As the blood is carried directly to the liver, absorbed food products may be immediately processed by liver cells; for example, glucose can be stored as glycogen. However, probably the main reason for the hepatic portal system is to allow the liver to break down bacterial metabolic toxins, generated in the lumen of the gut, before they enter the systemic circulation. If these toxins freely entered systemic blood, there would be a chronic, low-grade poisoning of all bodily organs.

CHAPTER 5

The lymphatic system

The lymphatic system consists of the lymphatic drainage vessels and other structures that contain lymphatic tissue. (Lymphatic tissue is also sometimes referred to as lymphoid tissue.)

Lymphatic drainage structures

Lymphatic capillaries

Most of the tissue fluid formed at the arterial end of the capillary is, as we have seen, reabsorbed back into the blood at the venous end of the capillary. However, along with tissue fluid, a few protein molecules also escape from the capillaries into the tissue spaces. If these large osmotic molecules were allowed to remain in the tissue fluid they would increase the osmotic potential, leading to an accumulation of water and resulting in oedema. Excess tissue fluid increases the diffusional distance between blood and tissue cells, and so reduces tissue viability. The mechanism that removes exuded proteins from the tissue fluid is the lymphatic drainage system. Once fluid has passed from the tissue spaces into a lymphatic vessel it is called lymph, or lymphatic fluid.

Unlike blood capillaries, the lymphatic capillaries are blind-ended; like blood capillaries, they are located in the tissue spaces. Lymphatic capillaries are highly permeable and will absorb excess tissue fluid and infecting bacteria, as well as proteins. Endothelial cells that compose the lymphatic capillary walls are separated by pores that allow fluid to enter. The cells also overlap slightly to form valves. As a lymphatic capillary fills with lymph, the pressure in the lumen will close the 'valves' in the wall of the capillary. This means fluid and other material is able to enter from the tissue spaces, but may not escape back out from the lymphatic capillaries.

One of the characteristics of cancer cells is that they no longer adhere to surrounding cells effectively. This means they may break away from their original location. These too may be absorbed by the lymphatic capillaries.

Afferent lymphatic vessels

Lymphatic capillaries drain into progressively larger lymphatic vessels. These lymphatic vessels have valves to ensure one-way flow of the lymphatic fluid (or lymph) away from the tissues and towards the

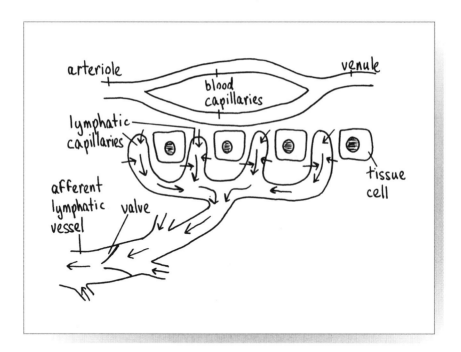

Diagram 5.1 Lymphatic capillaries are located between the cells and blood capillaries of the tissues. Once tissue fluid enters a lymphatic capillary it is referred to as lymphatic fluid. Arrows indicate direction of lymphatic fluid flow.

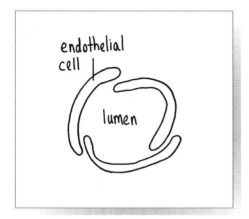

Diagram 5.2 Cross-section of an individual lymphatic capillary. Overlapping cells may 'flap' to allow larger objects to drain in with excess tissue fluids; they also act as valves.

lymph nodes. In this respect they function in a similar way to veins; however, they have more valves and thinner walls. As lymphatic vessels may drain bacteria from a site of tissue infection, it is sometimes possible to see 'tracking' of inflammation along the line of a lymphatic vessel. This is a classical clinical feature and may indicate spread of the infection.

Lymph nodes

These nodes are found throughout the body but are more common at particular sites such as the axilla and groin. There are also numerous internal lymph nodes in the thorax and abdomen. Lymph nodes are surrounded by a capsule composed of dense connective tissue. The capsule folds inwards forming trabeculae; these create spaces within the node referred to as sinuses. Throughout the node there is a network of reticular fibres. 'Reticulum' is Latin for 'net': these fibres form a three-dimensional network throughout the node. Several lymphatic vessels drain into a lymph node; these are referred to as afferent vessels. The lymphatic fluid then percolates through the node, and, because of the reticulum, bacteria get trapped.

Lymph nodes are also packed with white blood cells. Macrophages are able to phagocytose bacteria trapped in the reticular fibres. There are also numerous lymphocytes. T cells are able to recognize viruses and bacteria, and instruct B cells to produce antibodies. In addition, infection will trigger mitosis in B cells to produce many more B cells and plasma cells, capable of synthesizing large amounts of a specific antibody to combat an infection.

These functions mean the lymph nodes are able to trap and kill micro-organisms which are drained from infected tissue. They also function as an 'early warning' system for tissue infections. Infection may be recognized and an immune response commenced before any infection reaches the blood. Lymph nodes are able to do this because they are physiologically situated between the tissues and blood. Lymphatic fluid may only return to the blood once it has passed through a lymph node. When challenged by infection the lymph nodes swell, largely due to the proliferation of white blood cells. The correct term for this swelling is lymphadenopathy, but they are usually referred to as 'swollen glands'. Scientifically, lymph nodes are not glands because they do not produce an endocrine or exocrine produce.

In addition to filtering out foreign organisms, lymph nodes are able to filter cancer cells. It is then possible that a class of lymphocyte called an NK (natural killer) cells are active against the malignant cells (see page 248). Lymph nodes may therefore slow the spread of a cancer around the body.

If a lymphatic vessel is blocked, or several lymph nodes are surgically removed, this can lead to areas of localized oedema, as there is obstruction of normal lymphatic drainage.

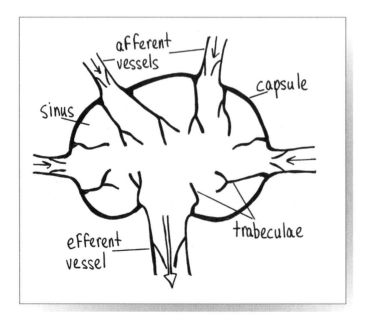

Diagram 5.3
A lymph node.

Efferent lymphatic vessels

The vessels carrying lymphatic fluid away from the lymph nodes are referred to as efferent. As the lymphatic fluid has been filtered through the lymph nodes it should be consistently sterile. Efferent lymphatic vessels join together to form larger drainage vessels called trunks. Trunks from the right side of the thorax, right arm and right side of the head and neck join to form the right lymphatic duct, which drains its contents directly into the right subclavian vein, located just under the clavicle.

Lymphatic trunks from both legs, abdomen, left side of the head, neck, thorax, and left arm all drain into the left lymphatic duct. This

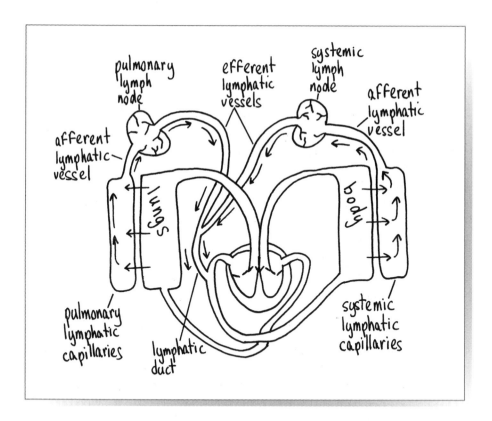

Diagram 5.4 Circulation of lymphatic fluid from the pulmonary and systemic lymphatic capillaries back into the systemic venous circulation. Arrows indicate direction of flow of lymphatic fluid.

is the main lymphatic duct in the body, and drains its fluid into the left subclavian vein. Two to three litres of fluid are drained back into the venous blood per day via the two lymphatic ducts. There is therefore a complete circulation of lymphatic fluid from the tissue spaces back into the venous blood.

Other lymphatic tissues

Lymphatic tissue is composed of fine reticular fibres that combine to form a connective tissue. These fine fibres often form a three-dimensional framework like scaffolding that can act as a support for other tissues and cells. The reticular fibres in lymphatic tissue support dense masses of white blood cells, particularly macrophages and lymphocytes. This lymphatic tissue is found not only in lymph nodes but also in several other structures.

Spleen

The spleen is located in the upper left area of the abdomen, just under the left costal margin (just below the ribs). In a similar way to lymph nodes filtering lymph, the spleen filters blood to ensure it remains sterile. There are two types of tissue in the spleen, referred to as red and white pulp.

White pulp is composed of lymphatic tissue and is full of lymphocytes and macrophages. These cells will kill any bacteria that have entered the blood. In addition, if micro-organisms are detected, this will trigger proliferation of defensive white cells. The sheer numbers of white cells in the spleen means that infections can often be eliminated before they have time to become established. This vital defensive role of the spleen is illustrated in people who had had their spleen removed (usually after a traumatic rupture). These people are no longer able to rapidly respond to a bacterial or viral challenge, and are at risk of sudden, overwhelming infection. Many take regular prophylactic antibiotics against this life-threatening possibility.

Red pulp carries out various functions related to red blood cells. It contains blood-filled spaces called sinusoids. Just as the spleen acts as a reservoir of white cells, it also holds a reserve of red cells. If there is haemorrhage, the spleen can contract and transfer blood from the sinusoids into the systemic circulation. In addition to this liquid blood, packed red blood cells from the red pulp may enter the systemic circulation if they are required. As a result, after a loss of blood the overall efficiency of the circulatory system can be rapidly restored. This allows a person to be able to fight or run effectively shortly after losing some blood, increasing the probability of survival after an injury, and it explains why people are able to return to work shortly after donating a unit of blood.

Various white blood cells including macrophages, lymphocytes and granulocytes, are also found in the red pulp. Macrophages in the red pulp phagocytose old and defective red blood cells, so the spleen is the main site of red cell breakdown, a process referred to as haemolysis.

Thymus gland

The thymus is located in the chest, posterior to the sternum. As well as the endocrine functions discussed in Chapter 3, the thymus is involved in the maturation of T lymphocytes. Immature, undifferentiated T cells divide in bone marrow and migrate to the thymus gland. Here they develop and differentiate into mature, immunocompetent T lymphocytes. Some of the T cells released from the thymus remain in the blood, but many travel to other areas of lymphoid tissue, such as the lymph nodes or spleen where they live. Most of the activity of the thymus in differentiation and maturation of T cells takes place in the few months before and after birth, although there is some ongoing activity in childhood. If the thymus gland is removed in adult life the function of the T lymphocytes is not seriously impaired.

Tonsils

These are collections of lymphoid tissue associated with the upper airway. This is a logical site for lymphoid tissue with reserves of leucocytes, as the airway is frequently exposed to bacteria and viruses in inhaled air. Tonsils are located under the moist epithelial lining of the pharynx and filter tissue fluid. This means they will filter any bacteria that have infected the epithelium or the tissue fluid beneath. Tonsils can become loaded with bacteria and severe tonsillitis may develop ('-itis' always means 'inflammation of'). In the past tonsils were surgically removed for repeated tonsillitis; however, it is now recognized

that tonsillitis is a sign that the tonsils are performing their immunological function. There are actually three collections of lymphatic tissue referred to as tonsils. These are in the nasopharynx, at the base of
the tongue and in the lateral walls of the oropharynx at the back of the
mouth. It is these tonsils in the oropharynx that people usually mean
when referring to 'tonsils'; their correct name is the palatine tonsils.

Diffuse lymphatic tissue

This form of lymphatic tissue is not surrounded by a capsule. In comparison, the spleen, lymph nodes and thymus are all compartmental-
ized by their own capsule. The appendix, attached to the caecum of
the large intestine, contains a lot of diffuse lymphatic tissue. In the
small intestine there are about 30 areas or patches of lymphoid tissue
located in the connective tissues of the ileum; these are referred to as
Peyer's patches. While small areas of diffuse lymphatic tissue can be
safely removed (such as in appendicectomy), collectively this lymphatic tissue is necessary to protect specific areas – and indeed the
whole body – from infections. In addition to these specific areas, small
amounts of lymphatic tissue are found in almost every organ of the
body.

CHAPTER 6

Blood

Components of blood

Blood contains two basic constituents. The first is the fluid component, referred to as plasma. Within the plasma floats the second component, the blood cells. Blood volume is normally made up of about
55% plasma and 45% cells. If an anticoagulant, such as heparin, is
added to a sample of blood, which is then centrifuged, all of the cells
will be forced to the bottom of the tube while the plasma remains
floating on top.

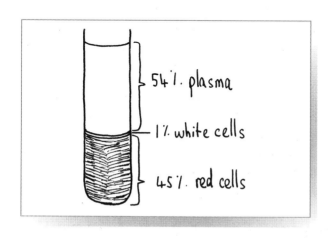

Diagram 6.1 Sample of
anticoagulated, centrifuged
blood to show the cellular
and plasma components.
Most of the cells are red but
there is a thin layer of white
cells just below the plasma.

Blood volumes

Blood volumes will clearly vary depending on the size of the person. At 6 months of age a baby will typically have a total of about 500 ml of blood; this will rise to a litre in a two-year-old. A 10-year-old may have about 2 litres and a 12-year-old a little over 3 litres. This has clear implications for the significance of blood loss in children; most adults can lose 500 ml of blood without any problems but in children this degree of loss could be fatal. Average size adults have a total of 5 litres of blood, with larger individuals having correspondingly more.

Plasma

Plasma is a yellowish fluid that is about 91% water. This keeps the blood fluid, to allow it to circulate around the body. The rest of the plasma is made up of various substances in solution; these include plasma proteins, nutrients and waste products.

Plasma proteins

Proteins are organic molecules made up of precise sequences of amino acids that are chemically bound together. There are three main plasma proteins: albumin, globulin and fibrinogen. Proteins are very large molecules and their presence is vital to generate plasma osmotic pressure. Without this osmotic property the blood would be unable to reabsorb tissue fluid. Albumin is the most common plasma protein and also generates most of the osmotic potential of plasma. The globulin proteins include the immunoglobulins (also called antibodies) that allow the body to fight off infections. Without these immune proteins we would probably die from the next virus or bacteria we pick up. Other globulin proteins act as carrier molecules that transport some hormones and minerals around the body. Fibrinogen is a vital clotting protein that allows blood to clot, to prevent bleeding.

As fats are not soluble in water they are transported around the body bound to plasma proteins. These combinations of fat and protein are termed lipoproteins and are soluble in water.

Nutrients and waste products

Plasma carries absorbed nutrients from the gut to all of the tissues of the body that need them; these include glucose, amino acids and vitamins. It also transports waste substances such as ammonia from the tissues to the liver, where this poisonous waste is converted into urea, which is much less toxic. Once formed, the urea is transported in solution from the liver to the kidneys for excretion.

Other plasma components and functions

Plasma is a carrying vehicle for a range of dissolved salts in ionic form; these include sodium, chloride, bicarbonate, potassium, phosphate, magnesium and calcium. Plasma also carries some dissolved gases such as carbon dioxide, nitrogen and a little oxygen. Most of the carbon dioxide transported by the blood is carried by the plasma. Plasma also transports the endocrine hormones from the gland to the target tissue.

Collectively the blood is also important in transporting heat around the body, helping to regulate body temperature. Heat from warm, metabolically active areas, such as the muscles and liver, must be transported away to prevent overheating. This warm blood can then be used to warm cooler areas such as the feet.

Blood is slightly alkaline. Arterial blood has a pH of 7.4, but venous blood is slightly more acidic with a normal pH of 7.35. This difference is caused by the increased volumes of carbon dioxide carried in the venous blood, some of which is carried as carbonic acid.

Blood cells

There are two main forms of blood cells, red cells – correctly termed erythrocytes – and white cells – correctly termed leucocytes.

Red cells

The function of the erythrocytes is to carry oxygen from lungs to tissues and carbon dioxide from tissues to lungs. The percentage of blood that is composed of red cells is termed the haematocrit; this may be lowered in some forms of anaemia. Red cells are biconcave discs; this shape provides a large surface area for gaseous exchange and also gives the cell flexibility. Some capillaries are so small the red cells have to squeeze through by deforming their shape. Red cells are about 7 micrometres in diameter (i.e. 7/1000 of a millimetre). Every cubic millimetre of blood contains about 5 million red blood cells.

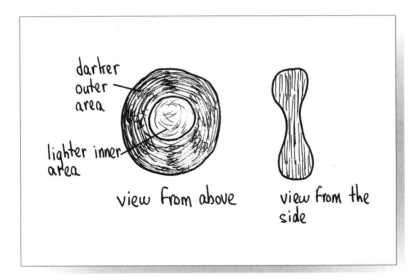

darker outer area

lighter inner area

view from above

view from the side

Diagram 6.2 Views of a red cell from above and the side. From above the outer thicker area of the cell appears to be darker red than the thinner, inner central area.

Blood is red because of the presence of the red cells. Erythrocytes are red because they contain a large pigmented protein molecule called haemoglobin. It is the haemoglobin that actually carries the oxygen. A single haemoglobin molecule can form a loose bond with four oxygen molecules. Although the haemoglobin molecule is large it is based on four atoms of iron. If there is no iron, haemoglobin cannot be synthesized. This is why iron deficiency will cause anaemia. (Anaemia means a reduced oxygen-carrying capacity of the blood.) Red blood cells are unique as they have no nucleus; this allows more space for carrying haemoglobin but also limits the life span of red cells to about 17 weeks.

In the lungs, dark red, deoxygenated haemoglobin will combine with oxygen to form bright red oxyhaemoglobin. In the capillaries of the tissues, the reverse will happen: oxyhaemoglobin will give up oxygen molecules and revert to deoxyhaemoglobin. The process may be summarized as follows:

In the lungs
Haemoglobin + oxygen → oxyhaemoglobin

In the tissues
Oxyhaemoglobin → haemoglobin + oxygen

Erythrocytes are formed from blood stem cells in the red bone marrow; this process is called erythropoiesis. (A stem cell is any cell that is capable of differentiation into other cell types.) Red bone marrow is found in the ends of long bones and in flat bones such as the sternum and pelvis. The regulation of erythropoiesis was discussed in the chapter on the endocrine system.

At the end of their lifespan, old red cells are phagocytosed by large cells called macrophages. This takes place mostly in the spleen, but also in the liver and bone marrow. Protein from the old red cells is broken down into amino acids and the iron is transported back to the bone marrow to be recycled. The coloured pigment from the haemoglobin is converted into a bile pigment called bilirubin, which is taken up by the liver and excreted into the small intestine in bile.

White cells

Leucocytes basically protect the body against disease and infection; this includes resistance to bacteria, viruses, worms, some toxins, and some cancers. They also unfortunately 'defend' the body against transplanted organs. This is because white cells are able to distinguish between 'self' and 'non-self' material, and will attack anything they perceive to be non-self. White cells are much less numerous than red cells; each cubic millimetre contains about 7 000 leucocytes.

There are two main forms of white cells. These are described according to the appearance of their cytoplasm. Some white cells have cytoplasm that appears granular, so this group are classified as granulocytes. Other white cells have cytoplasm that appears clear, with no granules; these are called agranulocytes ('a-' or 'an-' means 'without', so these cells are without granules). There are three types of granulocytes, called neutrophils, eosinophils and basophils (note all of the names of granulocytes end in '-phil'). There are only two main forms of agranulocytes, lymphocytes and monocytes. However, thrombocytes (platelets) are normally included in this group.

Neutrophils

Neutrophils are the most common form of leucocyte. Normally they compose 60–70% of the white cells in the blood. Most of the granules in the cytoplasm are fairly small and may be difficult to see under a light microscope. Granules in the cytoplasm contain lysozyme and a variety of other enzymes capable of digesting bacteria and other material during phagocytosis. The nucleus of a neutrophil has two to five lobes that are connected by fine threads; this is why neutrophils used to be called polymorphonuclear leucocytes ('poly-' means 'many' and 'morph-' relates to shape).

During an infection the number of neutrophils will increase significantly to help the body fight the causative micro-organism; this increase in number is called a neutrophil leucocytosis. As well as killing bacteria, neutrophils will also kill fungi and damaged or dead body cells. Neutrophils migrate out of inflamed blood vessels into areas where there is injury or infection to perform these immune functions. When body cells die (e.g. after injury) it is important that they are phagocytosed to remove them; if left, necrotic tissue forms an excellent habitat and food supply for infecting bacteria ('necrotic' means 'dead').

Eosinophils

These cells are often slightly larger than neutrophils, at about 13–15 micrometres; the cytoplasmic granules in eosinophils are larger than those found in neutrophils. Normally about 2–4% of the leucocytes in blood are eosinophils. The nucleus usually has two lobes, again joined by a thin thread. Eosinophils help the body fight infections of protozoa and larger parasites such as worms. They also are able to chemically neutralize histamines, which are involved in the generation of allergic responses. This is why eosinophil numbers increase in parasitic infections and allergic disorders. Many eosinophils migrate out of the blood to protect the tissues against potential infection, often where a body surface is exposed to the external environment. They are found associated with mucous membranes in the female reproductive tract, digestive organs and respiratory system.

Basophils

These cells are uncommon in the blood and only compose approximately 0.5% of leucocytes. The nucleus is irregular and lobed, but is often hard to see through the large, abundant granules in the cytoplasm. These granules contain histamine and heparin. The physiological role of basophils in the blood is unclear; however, most seem to enter the tissues where they remain localized. In the tissues they are called mast cells, where they are essential in the mediation of an inflammatory response (see page 237).

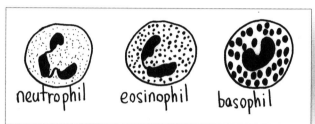

neutrophil   eosinophil   basophil

Diagram 6.3 The granulocytic leucocytes are neutrophils, eosinophils and basophils.

Lymphocytes

These are the most common form of agranulocytes; normally they comprise about 20–25% of circulating leucocytes. Lymphocytes may be classified as large or small. Large lymphocytes are the natural killer cells or NK cells and are able to kill body cells infected with viruses (see page 248).

Most of the lymphocytes are classified as small; they are about the same size as the red cells. The nucleus is large and spherical. Large numbers of lymphocytes can be found in lymphatic tissue, such as in the spleen, lymph nodes, tonsils and appendix. There are two main forms of small lymphocyte, called B and T. B lymphocytes mature in bone marrow and T lymphocytes mature in the thymus gland. The function of the B lymphocyte cell lines is the production of antibodies. An antibody is an immune protein, produced in response to the presence of a specific antigen. An antigen is something the immune system recognizes as foreign such as a measles virus.

There are three forms of T lymphocyte. These are called T helper cells, T cytotoxic cells and T suppressor cells. T helper cells 'help' B cells to produce antibodies. B cells will only produce antibodies when stimulated to do so by T helpers. Human immunodeficiency virus (HIV) attacks and kills T helper cells. This means they are unable to stimulate antibody production. Without the antibodies, immunodeficiency results, which can lead to acquired immunodeficiency syndrome (AIDS).

When B cells have produced enough antibody to deal with a particular infection, T suppressor cells inhibit B cell lines, and antibody production will be reduced. T cytotoxic cells have a range of defensive functions. They are able to detect and kill cells that are infected with viral particles. Although this strategy kills a body cell, it also kills the viruses in the cell, and so prevents them infecting further cells. Cytotoxic T cells are also able to detect and kill some cancer cells; it may be that malignant cells arise comparatively frequently, but are destroyed before they can divide to form a tumour. T killer cells will also directly attack foreign material such as parasites. (A fuller account of the role of leucocytes in immunity is given in Chapter 13.)

An increase in the number of lymphocytes is referred to as a lymphocytosis; this means more antibodies may be produced to counter any infection. The most common cause of this is a viral infection, but it also occurs in tuberculosis.

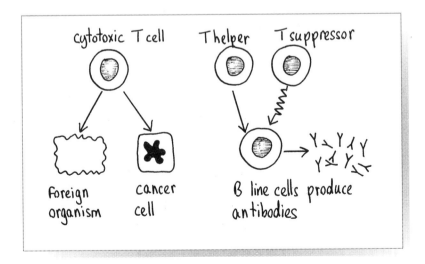

Diagram 6.4 Overview of the functions of the B and T lymphocytes.

Monocytes

Monocytes are large phagocytic cells; they may grow up to 20 micrometres in diameter. The nucleus is relatively large and is usually oval or kidney-shaped. They are able to migrate through capillary walls, by the process of amoeboid movement, to patrol the tissues. Amoeboid movement involves a flow of the cytoplasm within the cell membrane, moving the cell forward. Once in the tissues monocytes are usually referred to as macrophages. If any bacteria are encountered in the tissues they will rapidly be destroyed. 'Macro-' means 'big', and '-phage' means 'to eat', so by name and by function macrophages are literally 'big eaters'. Monocytes also produce pyrogens, which act on the hypothalamus to increase body temperature during infection. The number of monocytes is particularly likely to rise in chronic bacterial infections.

Thrombocytes

Thrombocytes or platelets are fragments of a type of white cell, and are essential for the process of blood clotting. If there is a deficiency of thrombocytes then blood clotting will be inhibited, resulting in haemorrhage and bruising. Lack of thrombocytes is termed thrombocytopenia.

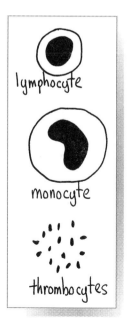

Diagram 6.5 The agranulocytic leucocytes are the lymphocytes, monocytes and thrombocytes.

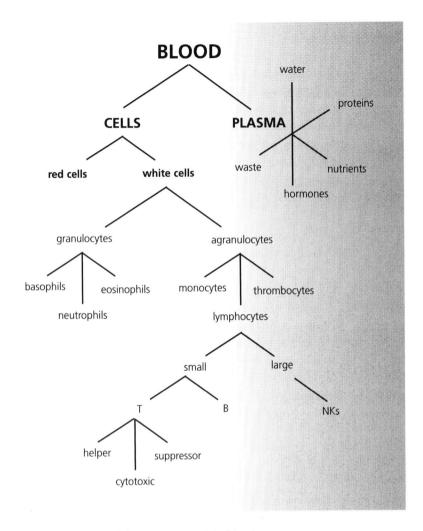

Table 6.1 Overview of the components of the blood.

Phagocytosis

Granulocytes and monocytes take part in the process of phagocytosis. This is the process whereby cells ingest and digest material the immune system has identified for destruction. Phagocytes are able to detect the presence of foreign material by a chemical recognition system (in other words they can 'smell' it). They are also able to recognize and phagocytose dead and damaged tissue cells. 'Phagocytosis' literally means 'cell-eating'; the following account describes how a phagocyte eats a group of bacteria.

When the bacteria are detected the phagocyte moves towards them; phagocytes are capable of an independent form of locomotion called chemotaxis that uses amoeboid movement. Once the phagocyte arrives next to the bacteria, it carries on moving towards them. The result of this is that the bacteria become engulfed by the cell membrane and cytoplasm of the phagocyte. Eventually the bacteria are completely enclosed in the cytoplasm of the phagocyte, within a vacuole composed of external cell membrane. After this, lysosomes move towards the newly formed vacuole. Lysosomes are specialist organelles that contain digestive enzymes such as lysozyme. When the membranes surrounding the lysosomes and the vacuole come into contact they fuse, allowing the digestive enzymes to pour on to the trapped bacteria, which will then be digested into constituent carbohydrates and amino and fatty acids. These products of digestion are then absorbed by the phagocyte and surrounding cells as nutrients. A few breakdown products from the bacteria which are not absorbed are ejected from the cell.

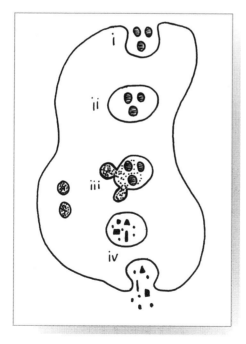

Diagram 6.6 Diagram of the sequential stages of phagocytosis.

(i) After moving towards the bacteria they are ingested: the phagocyte 'eats' them.

(ii) Bacteria are now isolated in a vacuole.

(iii) Lysosomes move towards the bacteria-containing vacuole and the membranes merge. This pours digestive enzymes from the lysosomes onto the bacteria, which are then digested.

(iv) Products of digestion that are not absorbed are excreted from the cell.

ABO Rhesus system of blood grouping

People may be one of the four possible major blood groups. They may be A, B, AB or O. In addition to these four groups there is a further group called the Rhesus factor. This is an additional factor that a person may or may not have in addition to being A, B, AB or O. An individual may therefore be A Rhesus positive or negative, B Rhesus positive or negative, AB Rhesus positive or negative or O Rhesus positive or negative.

The blood group a person has depends on the nature of their red cells, which is in turn genetically programmed. Blood groups are determined by protein-based structures located on the external membranes of the red cells.

These grouping molecules are specific proteins which possess a particular molecular shape and are referred to as antigens. Someone is blood group A if they have A antigens on their red cells. In blood group B the person has B antigens on the surface of their red cells. The presence of group AB antigens on the surface of the red cells means the individual would be group AB. People with group O have no antigens on the surface of their red cells. In fact, O is a corruption of zero so really the blood groups should be A, B, AB and zero but we have changed this to O. So a person with blood group O actually has no ABO grouping antigens on the surface of their red cells. The Rhesus factor is also an antigen, which is simply either present or absent on the surface of the red blood cells.

Use of the term 'antigen' in reference to blood groups often causes confusion because an antigen is something the body recognizes as foreign. Clearly the body should not recognize its own proteins as foreign. However, this physiology was first worked out with reference to blood transfusions, so the term antigen is used with reference to the recipient of donated blood. The recipient's immune systems would recognize the group-defining proteins on donated red cells as antigenic if they were from an incompatible group.

In addition to the antigens which determine blood group there are also associated antibodies present or absent in the plasma of particular blood groups. These antibodies are to all of the ABO antigens the individual does not possess, so if a person is blood group A they will have antibodies to antigen B in their plasma. If a person is blood group B they will have antibodies to antigen A in their plasma. In blood group AB they will be no antibodies in the plasma, and if a person is blood group O they will have A and B antibodies in their plasma.

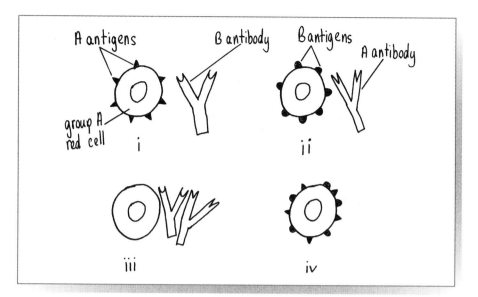

Diagram 6.7 The ABO blood grouping system.

(i)   Blood group A has A antigens on the red cells and B antibodies in the plasma.

(ii) Blood group B has B antigens on the red cells and antibody A in the plasma.

(iii) Blood group O has no (zero) antigens on the red cells and both antibodies A and B in the plasma.

(iv) Blood group AB has A and B antigens on the red cells but no antibodies in the plasma.

An antibody is a protein found in the blood that will bind to its specific reciprocal antigen. This means an A antibody will bind to an A antigen if the two come into contact. Therefore, if a person with group A blood gives some blood to a person with group B blood, the A antibodies in the recipient's plasma will bind to the A antigens on the donor's red cells. This will cause many of the donated red cells to clump together in a process called agglutination.

This is a potentially life-threatening complication of blood transfusion. It is therefore necessary that there are no antibodies in a recipient's plasma to the antigens of the donated blood. If a person with group B blood donates blood to a person with group A blood then the B antibodies in the recipient's plasma will bind to the B antigens on the given red cells. This will cause agglutination (i.e. clumping) of the donated cells with the recipient's antibodies. Clumps of red cells will, over time, be broken down in the process of haemolysis; this is why transfusion mismatches are sometimes referred to as transfusion haemolytic reactions.

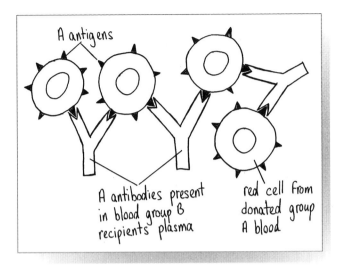

Diagram 6.8 In this case group A blood has been given to a group B recipient by mistake. The result is that the A antibodies in the recipient's plasma bind to the A antigens on the surface of the donor's red cells. This results in agglutination.

In theory, each blood group can give to people with the same group as themselves, because they will share the same antibodies. Because people with group AB blood have no antibodies in their plasma they can, in ABO terms, receive blood from anyone. As they have no antibodies in their plasma, there will be no antibodies to bind to donated antigens, therefore there will be no agglutination. A person with group O blood can give blood to any other person because their blood contains no antigens. This means that whatever antibodies may be present in the recipient's plasma there will be no agglutination of donated cells. These principles explain why AB is sometimes referred to as the universal recipient and O as the universal donor.

Recipients	Donors			
	A	B	AB	O
A	✓	X	X	✓
B	X	✓	X	✓
AB	✓	✓	✓	✓
O	X	X	X	✓

Table 6.2 Summary of which donated blood may be given to which recipients in the ABO system.

Rhesus factor

The second common blood grouping uses the Rhesus (Rh) factor, so called because it was first discovered in Rhesus monkeys. Rhesus factor is in addition to the ABO groups. This factor is simply present or absent on the red cells. Unlike the ABO system there are no naturally occurring antibodies in the plasma; however, antibodies may develop in a Rhesus negative individual if they are exposed to Rhesus positive blood.

Recipients who are Rhesus negative should therefore only receive Rhesus negative blood. If they were to be given Rhesus positive blood there would be no reaction on the first occasion; however, the introduction of Rhesus antigens would cause the recipient to produce Rhesus factor antibodies. This means if the patient were to be given Rhesus positive blood on a second occasion, the new Rhesus factor antibodies would bind to the donated Rhesus factor antigen, leading to agglutination. Therefore Rhesus negative recipients may only receive Rhesus negative blood. In theory, however, Rhesus positive patients may receive Rhesus negative blood, as the red cells contain no antigens.

Once the Rhesus factor is taken into account it means that O negative is the universal donor and AB positive the universal recipient. The Rhesus factor is sometimes referred to as the D factor. This is because the most active component of the Rhesus factor antigen is termed the D factor.

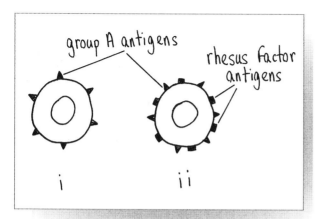

Diagram 6.9 The Rhesus factor is present or absent.
(i) Group A red cell which is Rhesus negative.
(ii) Group A red cell which is Rhesus positive.

Rhesus factor incompatibility in pregnancy and neonates

This problem arises as a result of the genetic transmission of Rhesus factor from parents to children. When a mother is Rh-negative and the father is Rh-positive there is a chance the baby will be Rh-positive. There will be a 50% or a 100% chance of a baby being Rh-positive, depending on the genetic makeup of the father.

In Rhesus incompatibility, the mother will develop Rhesus antibodies if there is blood-to-blood contact with her Rh-positive baby. Mixing of maternal and baby blood may occur during birth. The Rhesus factor in the baby's blood will act as an antigen in the circulation of the mother, causing her to produce Rhesus antibodies. This does not usually affect the baby during the first pregnancy; however, during subsequent pregnancies the mother will already possess antibodies to the Rh factor. This can result in her antibodies attacking the baby's blood, leading to a condition called haemolytic disease of the newborn. Affected babies have a reduced oxygen-carrying capacity of the blood and are jaundiced, due to the presence of red cell breakdown products such as bilirubin.

This complication should now be prevented by the administration of an Anti-D injection, given to the mother after the birth of every baby. These injected D antibodies quickly destroy (mop up) any Rh-positive baby cells in the mother's blood. The result of this intervention is that Rh-positive cells are not present in the maternal circulation for long enough to stimulate the mother's immune system to produce antibodies to the Rhesus factor.

Haemostasis

This describes the process whereby bleeding stops when a blood vessel is ruptured; the aim is to prevent ongoing blood loss. Bleeding may occur from any of the blood vessels, i.e. haemorrhage may be arterial, venous or capillary. Haemostasis may be considered under three headings: vascular spasm, platelet plugging and the coagulation cascade.

Vascular spasm

In vascular spasm the smooth muscle of a blood vessel wall constricts after being damaged or cut. As a blood vessel constricts, the diameter of the lumen is reduced, lessening the blood loss from the cut or dam-aged vessel. This mechanism is aided by cold and inhibited by heat. One reason why some severely injured soldiers survived in the Falklands war is that the cold conditions aided vascular shut-down, which prevented life-threatening blood loss.

Platelet plugging

The second stage is referred to as platelet plugging. When the lining of a blood vessel is damaged substances are released which activate platelets making them become very sticky; this means that the platelets adhere to the injury to form a temporary plug. This is suffi-cient to block small damaged vessels and prevent capillary bleeding.

Coagulation cascade

The third phase is referred to as the coagulation cascade; this is the actual process of blood clotting. There are twelve factors responsible for this, denoted by the relevant Roman numerals. Overall, the process converts liquid blood into a semi-solid mass that forms a plug over the injury; once formed, this can stay in position for several days.

Any cascade consists of a series of pre-synthesized components in an inactive form. In the case of the clotting cascade these components are present in the blood. A stimulus triggers off the first reaction in a cascade, which then triggers the second and so on. The activation of the final component of a cascade normally brings about a significant physiological change, in this case blood clotting. The advantage of having numerous steps to a cascade is that the process can be inhibited at any stage by negative feedback activity (see page 245 for another example of a cascade).

The process of clotting starts when factor XII (also called Hageman factor after the person it was discovered in) comes into contact with collagen in the damaged wall of a blood vessel. Factor XII is a plasma protein which is normally present in plasma, but in an inactive form. It is the contact with collagen that activates factor XII causing it to function as an enzyme.

Once activated, factor XII in turn activates further factors which eventually cause the inactive plasma protein called prothrombin to be broken down into thrombin, a much smaller protein. Factors derived from platelets and calcium ions are required for some of the steps in the process. Prothrombin is continually used for blood clotting throughout the body so must be continually synthesized in the liver. Vitamin K is necessary for the formation of prothrombin and fibrinogen. This is why patients with liver failure or vitamin K deficiency may suffer from haemorrhagic features. Warfarin also acts by inhibition of vitamin K; this leads to lack of clotting factors in the plasma and so will cause anticoagulation.

Once formed, thrombin acts on the large, soluble plasma protein called fibrinogen and converts it into the insoluble protein, fibrin. Fibrin consists of long sticky threads that form the reticulum of the blood clot. The fibrin strands initially cover and reinforce the platelet plug. They will also stick to the cut or damaged edges of the blood vessel forming a network over the injury; blood cells and other components of the plasma are caught in the fibrin network which holds everything together forming a blood clot.

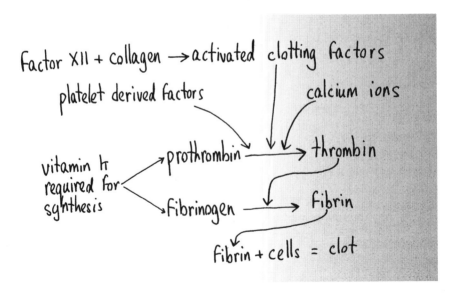

Table 6.3 The principal stages in blood clotting.

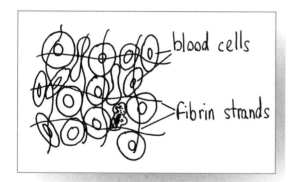

Diagram 6.10 A blood clot forms when blood cells adhere to sticky strands of fibrin.

Breakdown of blood clots

A blood clot is a temporary measure to prevent blood loss. As the tissues regenerate to heal the initial injury, the blood clot needs to be removed.

When a blood clot is formed, a plasma protein called plasminogen is trapped in the clot along with other plasma proteins. Damaged tissues and vascular endothelium release a substance called tissue plasminogen activator. Over the course of a few days this will progressively convert the trapped plasminogen into plasmin. Plasmin acts as a protein-digesting (proteolytic) enzyme which breaks down the fibrin threads and so dissolves the blood clot. Plasmin is also sometimes called fibrinolysin ('-lysis' means 'to break down').

CHAPTER 7

Respiration

Respiration describes breathing and the utilization of oxygen within the cells of the body. Traditionally the term external respiration has been used to describe the processes of breathing, while internal respiration relates to how oxygen is used in the cells of the body to generate energy.

Structures of the respiratory system

Nose and mouth

Air passing through the nose is warmed; this is achieved by contact with the internal nasal passages, which are well perfused with warm blood. Warming the air prevents the lower airways being chilled. As the linings of the nasal passages are moist, air passing through the nose is also humidified; this protects the lower airways from possible drying effects of air. The mucus lining, in combination with nasal hair, has the effect of filtering air passing through the nose, removing foreign bodies such as small insects. Strangely, the sense of smell provides much of the sensation of taste (which is why food seems to lose much of its taste when we have a cold). Smell also alerts us to the dangers of poisonous gases and bad food.

The nasal septum divides the nasal cavity into left and right sides (a septum is a structure which divides). The back part of the septum is made of bony tissue and the front part of more flexible cartilage. Young babies breathe exclusively through the nose; this means if their noses are blocked for any reason they will asphyxiate. The mouth can increase the size of the airway opening to increase the volumes of air that can be inhaled.

Sinuses

These are small air-filled cavities in some of the frontal bones of the skull. They are lined with mucus that drains into the nasal cavity via small passages. The function of the sinuses seems to be to lighten the weight of the skull and to give resonance to the voice. Infection may spread from the nose into the sinuses, giving rise to the common painful condition of sinusitis.

Pharynx

This is the passage that connects the back of the nose and mouth with the trachea and oesophagus. It is composed of three sections: the nasopharynx is behind the nasal cavity; below this is the oropharynx behind the mouth. The lower section is called the laryngopharynx, which leads down to the oesophagus and trachea.

Larynx

The larynx extends from the laryngopharynx to the start of the trachea. Because the structure is mostly composed of cartilage it can easily be felt in the neck, where it is commonly referred to as the 'Adam's apple'. As the larynx contains the vocal cords (more correctly known as vocal folds) it is often referred to as the 'voice box'. The vocal cords are elastic ligaments that can be tightened or relaxed. As air passes over the cords they vibrate, producing sound. The vibrations can be controlled by regulating how tight or relaxed the cords are. Tight cords will produce high-pitched sounds, and when they are more relaxed the pitch of the sound will be lower. If we vibrate the folds at a rate of 256 hertz (cycles per second) this will produce a musical middle C.

Epiglottis

During swallowing food must pass over the entrance of the larynx to enter the oesophagus. The opening into the larynx is called the glottis and just above this is a sheet of elastic cartilage called the epiglottis. In order to allow movement, the epiglottis is attached to the cartilage of the larynx at the front forming a type of hinge. During swallowing, the free posterior portion of the epiglottis forms a seal over the glottis. This seal prevents a food bolus entering into the airway by providing a pathway over the top of the epiglottis into the oesophagus. If this fails to work, food may enter the trachea (going down the 'wrong way') causing choking (the most common cause of choking is talking and eating at the same time).

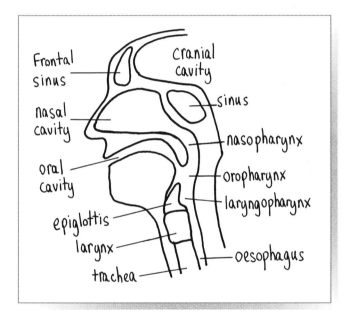

Diagram 7.1 Structures of the upper respiratory tract.

Trachea

The trachea, or windpipe, is about 10 cm long and extends from the bottom of the larynx to the bifurcation into the left and right main bronchus. It is vital that the trachea is patent at all times as it is the only way air can enter and exit the lungs. To ensure it is kept open, the walls contain incomplete rings of cartilage. These rings of cartilage are rigid to prevent collapse, and they are incomplete to allow the smooth passage of food down the oesophagus, which is immediately behind the trachea.

Diagram 7.2
Cross-section of the
trachea and oesophagus.

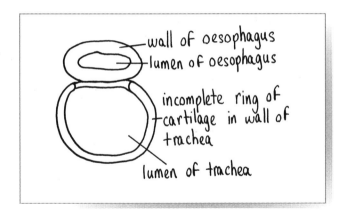

- wall of oesophagus
- lumen of oesophagus

incomplete ring of cartilage in wall of trachea

lumen of trachea

Respiratory lining

The lumen of the trachea and other respiratory passages are lined with a columnar mucous membrane. Numerous goblet cells are present in the trachea and bronchi; these produce mucus that lines the internal surfaces. Inhaled particles, such as dust or aggregates of bacteria, stick to the mucus and are then wafted up towards the trachea by cilia. The cilia are microscopic hair-like projections from cell surfaces that waft the mucus in one direction to help to clear foreign material and bacteria from the lungs. Once the mucus is in the trachea it may be coughed up, by a blast of air, through the vocal cords into the back of the mouth; from here it may be spat out or swallowed.

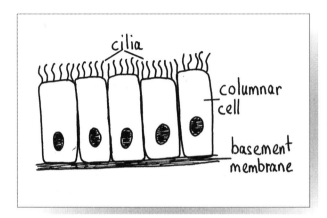

cilia

columnar cell

basement membrane

Diagram 7.3
Ciliated columnar
epithelium. Cilia waft mucus
towards the trachea, away
from the alveoli.

Left and right bronchus

The trachea divides into the left and right primary bronchus, one entering each lung (the primary bronchi are also called the main bronchi). The right primary bronchus is more a continuation of the trachea than the left, which branches off at a greater angle. This means that if a foreign body is accidentally inhaled it usually enters the right bronchus.

Bronchial tubes

Each primary bronchus divides into secondary bronchi, also referred to as lobar bronchi, because one enters each lobe of the lung. The right

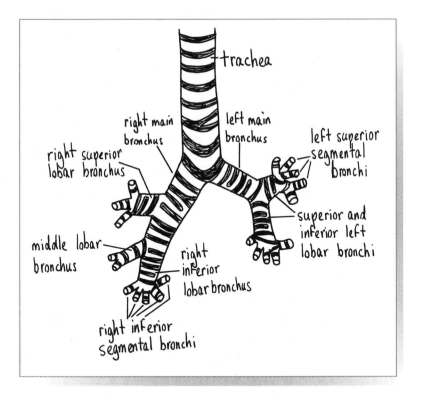

Diagram 7.4 The large structures of the bronchial tree: one trachea; two primary (main) bronchi; five secondary (lobar) bronchi; and twenty tertiary (segmental) bronchi. Two left lobar bronchi branch into five segmental bronchi each. The right superior lobar bronchus branches into three segmental bronchi, the right middle into two and the right inferior into five.

lung is composed of three lobes while the left has two. Secondary bronchi in turn divide into smaller tertiary bronchi. These are also referred to as segmental bronchi because one enters each segment of a lobe. Each lung has a total of 10 segments with 10 corresponding segmental bronchi.

Bronchioles

As the bronchial tree continues to divide into smaller airways, the rings of cartilage are lost. After 12 to 16 divisions the diameter is reduced to 1 mm or less and the tubes are referred to as bronchioles. These airways are still lined with mucus-secreting columnar epithelium with cilia, to waft mucus upwards towards the trachea. In turn the bronchioles branch into still smaller terminal bronchioles; however, even in these smaller structures the walls are still too thick to allow any gaseous exchange to occur between the air and blood.

Terminal bronchioles further divide into respiratory bronchioles that terminate in the alveolar air sacs. The walls of the respiratory bronchioles have a few alveoli in their walls to increase internal surface area. Gaseous exchange between the air and blood only takes place in the microscopic respiratory bronchioles and alveoli. Overall, the bronchial tree forms a fractal pattern with each smaller pattern duplicating the larger one it has branched from. This means that each terminal area of the tree receives equal volumes of fresh inhaled air and is able to exhale air equally freely.

Bronchial diameters

The airways are able to dilate and constrict under the control of the autonomic nervous system. All of the airways contain smooth muscle fibres in their walls; when these contract bronchoconstriction will result and when they relax there will be bronchodilation. During a 'fight or flight' reaction more oxygen is required for muscular activity. This is why sympathetic stimulation will relax the smooth muscle, leading to airway dilation. This will also allow more carbon dioxide, produced by increased skeletal muscle activity, to be exhaled. If the airways were dilated all of the time, infection would be able to penetrate into the lungs more readily. This is why when an individual is at rest the parasympathetic nervous system constricts the airways to reduce their lumen. If irritants are inhaled there will also be a reflex bronchoconstriction to limit the amount that is able to enter the lungs.

Alveoli

Respiratory bronchioles terminate in groups of alveoli termed alveolar sacs. Alveoli have very thin walls, and 90% of the surface area is composed of squamous cells. The remaining 10% of the alveolar wall is composed of septal cells that produce surfactant; this substance reduces the surface tension of the water that moistens internal surfaces of the air sacs. It is vital that the internal respiratory surfaces are moist, as oxygen will not diffuse into a dry surface. However, the reduction in surface tension is also essential to prevent the walls of the alveoli sticking together after expiration. Premature babies often lack surfactant and this leads to the disorder called respiratory distress syndrome (RDS). Because the alveoli are the site of gaseous exchange the walls of the alveolar sacs are folded into structures which resemble hollow bunches of grapes. Infolding greatly increases the respiratory surface area to about 143 m^2 in total (71.5 m^2 per lung). There are about 300 million alveoli in the two lungs. Elastic fibres support the walls of the alveoli, giving them natural elasticity.

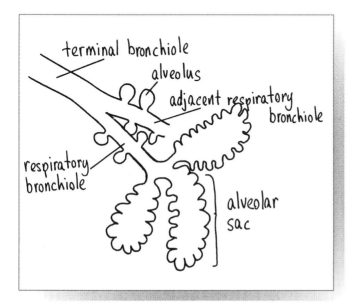

Diagram 7.5
A group of alveoli branching from a respiratory bronchiole.

The lungs

Lungs are very light organs as the alveoli are mostly filled with air. This is why lung fields appear dark on X-ray films. Because they do not contain a large mass of tissue, most of the X-rays pass straight through. The left lung is composed of two lobes, each lobe consisting of five segments. These segments are correctly referred to as bronchopulmonary segments. The right lung is in three lobes. The superior lobe contains three segments, the middle lobe two and the inferior lobe five. This division of the lungs into lobes has an important role in compartmentalizing some infections. For example, in lobar pneumonia the infection is usually confined to a single lobe. (Pneumonia means infection of the lung tissue.)

Diagram 7.6

Overall structure and lobes of the lungs.

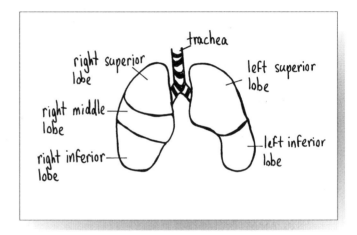

Blood and lymphatic vessels

Deoxygenated blood is transported to the lungs via the pulmonary arteries. Oxygenated blood returns to the heart via the pulmonary veins. Each segment of the lung is individually supplied with blood via a pulmonary segmental artery and drained by a segmental vein. Each segment also has its own lymphatic drainage system. Like the bronchial tree, the arterial and venous pulmonary vessels also form a fractal pattern. A fractal arrangement ensures all areas of the lungs receive an equal supply of blood and are equally drained. This means there are three superimposed fractal trees in the lungs: bronchial, arterial and venous.

Mechanical ventilation

Skeletal structures associated with respiration

The lungs are surrounded with bones that provide protection against damage from outside trauma. Protection from the back is provided by the thoracic vertebral column. However, the bony structures are also essential to facilitate the mechanical process of breathing. The breastbone or sternum is the flat bone in the front of the chest. There are 12 pairs of ribs, which form a cage-like structure around the lungs; the first 10 pairs of ribs are connected to the sternum via costal cartilage ('costal' means 'to do with ribs'). Men and women, of course, both have the same number of ribs.

Muscles associated with respiration

The diaphragm is a sheet of skeletal muscle that divides the thoracic and abdominal cavities. When the muscle of the diaphragm is at rest the structure is domed upwards. Contraction causes it to flatten downwards. The ribs are joined together by sheets of intercostal muscles that follow the line of the ribs around the chest. (These are the muscles you eat if you have barbecue spare ribs.) There are two sets of intercostal muscles, the external and internal. The diaphragm and the intercostal muscles are referred to as the primary respiratory muscles. In addition, there are some accessory muscles, attached to the sternum and upper ribs, that aid the expansion of the thorax during more vigorous respiratory activity.

Inspiration

To facilitate inspiration the diaphragm contracts, causing it to move down and flatten. At the same time the external intercostal muscles pull the rib cage up and out. Both of these movements result in an increase in the volume of the thoracic cavity. Because the volume of the thorax is increased the pressure of air left inside the thorax in the lungs is reduced. Gases will always move from areas of high pressure to areas of lower pressure. As there is a pressure reduction in the thorax, air moves in from the outside to equalize the pressures between the

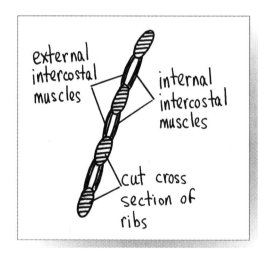

external
intercostal
muscles

internal
intercostal
muscles

cut cross
section of
ribs

Diagram 7.7 A section of chest wall showing the ribs and intercostal muscles.

atmosphere and the reduced pressure inside the lungs. So, in inspiration, when air is sucked into the lungs the process is one of negative pressure ventilation. This contrasts with artificial respiration, in which air is actively blown into the lungs, so-called positive pressure ventilation. The increase in the volume of air in the lungs stretches the elastic tissues and smooth muscle associated with the walls of the bronchioles and alveoli. This is analogous to blowing up a balloon.

Expiration

During expiration, the smooth muscle and elastic tissue in the walls of the bronchioles and alveoli recoils. This reduces the volume of these structures and so increases the pressure of the air they contain. This is analogous to releasing the pressure on the neck of a balloon; as the elastic walls of the balloon recoil, the pressure is increased so air is blown out. These properties mean that overall the lungs are elastic – they passively recoil, which increases the air pressure in the lungs as a whole, and thus air is blown out.

To assist this process the diaphragm relaxes and so moves up; the external intercostal muscles also relax which allows the ribs to fall down and in. The movement of the diaphragm up, and of the ribs down and in, reduces the volume of the thoracic cavity. Because the volume is reduced the pressure is increased. This means the pressure inside the lungs is now greater than in the external atmosphere so air is blown out of the lungs. From this it can be seen that while inspiration is an active, muscular process, expiration is a passive process caused by elastic recoil and muscle relaxation. During vigorous respiration the process of expiration needs to be faster, so the process is aided by contraction of the internal intercostal muscles. These pull the ribs down and in rapidly and actively. These muscles are also essential during periods of increased airway resistance. This happens during an asthmatic attack, when the bronchial lumens are narrowed and air needs be forced out against the increased resistance.

Monitoring the rate, depth and rhythm of breathing is a fundamental aspect of nursing observations. One respiration consists of one inspiration followed by one expiration. These may be counted by observation of chest movements and should be recorded over a period of one minute. The respiratory rhythm should be regular and a rate of about 12 per minute is normal during periods of rest. In emergency situations assessment of the airway is always a first priority; if we put our ear near the patient's mouth and look down at their chest we are able to 'look, listen and feel' the breathing.

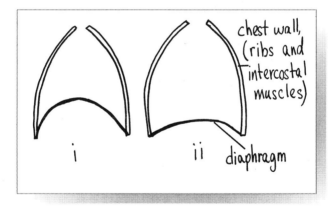

Diagram 7.8

(i) At the end of expiration the ribs are down and in and the diaphragm is domed upwards.

(ii) To facilitate inspiration the ribs move up and out while the diaphragm flattens.

Pleural membranes

There are two pleural membranes surrounding the lungs. First, the visceral is the inner membrane; one visceral membrane surrounds the surface of each lung. Second, the parietal is the outer membrane lining the inside of the thoracic cavity; this pleural membrane also lines the superior surface of the diaphragm. Between these two membranes there is a negative pressure of about –4 mm of mercury, which has the effect of sucking the two membranes together. This means the area between the two pleural membranes is only a potential space. (A potential space is when two membranes are immediately adjacent to each other but not directly connected by tissue; the result of this is that a space could be created should something be introduced between the two layers.)

When the ribs move up and out while the diaphragm moves down, the parietal pleural membrane moves with these structures as it is adherent to them and invaginates them. Because there is a negative pressure between the parietal and visceral pleural membrane, the visceral pleural membrane is drawn up and out with the chest wall, and down with the diaphragm. As the visceral pleural membrane is adherent to the surface of the lungs and invaginates the surface of the lung tissue, the lungs expand with their visceral pleural membrane. This is why the lungs expand with the chest wall and diaphragm.

The visceral pleural membrane expands because of the suction of the visceral pleural membrane onto the parietal pleural membrane. Therefore, if any air gets into the potential pleural space (that is, between the visceral and parietal pleural membranes), through a stab wound, for example, the negative pressure will be lost, movement of

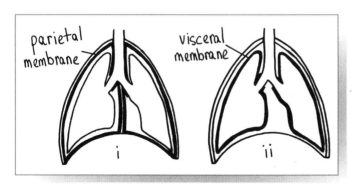

parietal membrane

visceral membrane

i

ii

Diagram 7.9
(i) Parietal pleural membranes.
(ii) Visceral pleural membranes.

the parietal pleural membrane will then no longer result in movement of the visceral pleural membrane and the lung would collapse. This condition is known as pneumothorax and requires immediate emergency medical treatment. Fortunately, there is usually time to transfer such patients to hospital as the two lungs are each surrounded by a separate visceral and parietal pleural membrane; this means one penetrating injury only results in the collapse of one lung and it is possible to survive on the other single lung for a time.

Respiratory volumes

During normal, quiet breathing, about 500 ml of air moves in and out of the respiratory system per breath. The volume of inspired or expired air is referred to as the tidal volume. During exercise the tidal volumes will increase. The minute volume of respiration can be calculated by multiplying the tidal volume by the minute respiratory rate. If this rate is 12 and the tidal volume is 500 ml the minute volume will be 6 litres. During inhalation, not all of the air reaches the respiratory surfaces. About 150 ml is left in the nose, pharynx, larynx and bronchial passages, and is referred to as the 'dead air volume'; the space occupied by

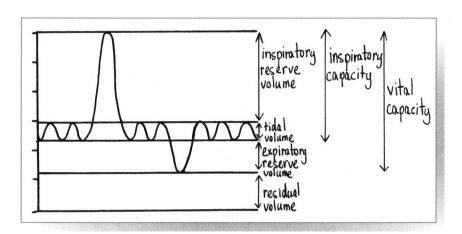

Diagram 7.10 The range of approximate adult normal respiratory volumes in mls:

Inspiratory reserve	3 100	Tidal volume at rest	500
Expiratory reserve	1 200	Residual	1 000
Inspiratory capacity	3 600	Vital capacity	4 800

this volume of air is called the 'dead space'. The presence of dead space means only about 350 ml of fresh atmospheric air reaches the lungs as a result of inspiration at rest.

It is possible to increase the tidal volume intake of air by about 3 litres per breath; this additional reserve volume is termed the inspiratory reserve volume. Likewise it is possible to breath out more air than normal; this is called the expiratory reserve volume. However, even with full strained expiration there will always be at least 1 litre of air left in the lungs, the residual volume. The combination of the expiratory reserve volume and the inspiration reserve is termed the vital capacity. The total lung capacity is normally about 6 litres.

Gaseous exchange

The right ventricle contracts, ejecting blood through the pulmonary arterial valve into the pulmonary artery. The pulmonary artery subdivides into smaller arteries and ultimately, via arterioles, into the capillaries that surround the alveoli. Because the blood in the right ventricle has returned from the body it is deoxygenated: the blood in the pulmonary arterial system is low in oxygen and relatively high in carbon dioxide. The walls of the pulmonary capillaries and the walls of

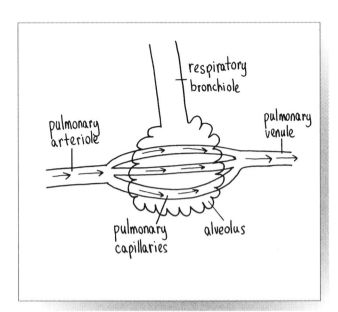

Diagram 7.11
Pulmonary capillaries surround the alveoli. Arrows indicate direction of blood flow.

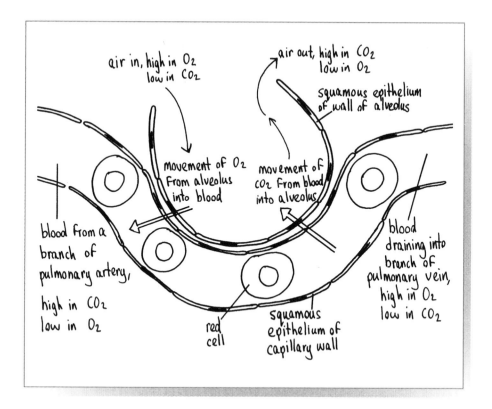

Diagram 7.12
The walls of the capillaries and alveoli
are both composed of squamous cells.
This means the diffusional distance
between the air and blood is small, in
order to allow gaseous exchange.

the alveoli are both very thin, made of squamous epithelial cells, which
means the diffusional distance between air and blood is small. Also, the
lining of the alveoli is moist, allowing oxygen to diffuse into the surface.
Oxygen is therefore able to diffuse through the cell walls of the alveoli
and capillaries into the blood and, vice versa, carbon dioxide from the
blood into the alveoli. This means that the blood leaving the lungs to
return to the left side of the heart via the pulmonary veins is now high
in oxygen and low in carbon dioxide.

Transport of gases in blood

Approximately 98.5% of the oxygen absorbed into the blood is transported by haemoglobin molecules in the red cells. The remaining 1.5% is transported in solution in plasma. These figures explain why people who have lost a lot of blood require blood transfusions. Replacement of fluids alone will result in an inadequate ability to transport oxygen from lungs to tissues. Oxygen saturation monitoring is now common in clinical practice and this reveals that blood is normally 98–99% saturated. This indicates how efficiently oxygen is absorbed by the blood passing through the lungs.

Carbon dioxide (CO_2) is carried from tissues to the lungs in three ways. First, about 7% of the total CO_2 is simply carried in solution after dissolving into the plasma. Second, a further 23% combines with haemoglobin and is transported in red cells. Third, 70% forms bicarbonate ions (HCO_3^-) in combination with water in the plasma. In the lungs these ions dissociate back into CO_2 which then diffuses into the alveoli. A small amount is also transferred in the form of carbonic acid, H_2CO_3; this is why blood pH rises if there is retention of CO_2.

Composition of air

Atmospheric air is a mixture of approximately 21% oxygen, 78% nitrogen and 0.04% carbon dioxide; several other trace inert gases are also present such as argon, helium and neon. The amount of water in the air is dependent on the ambient humidity. Because oxygen is absorbed into the blood, expired air contains about 16% oxygen. The presence of this oxygen in expired air is why exhaled-air mouth-to-mouth ventilation may be used to keep a patient oxygenated for a short time. As carbon dioxide is excreted from the lungs, the proportion rises to around 4% of the exhaled air volume. There is an equilibrium between nitrogen in the air and in solution in plasma, so the proportion of this inert gas in inhaled and exhaled air is the same.

Regulation of respiration

Respiration is controlled by the respiratory centre located in the medulla oblongata, the lowest part of the brain stem. These cells seem to coordinate a natural rhythm that generates nerve impulses to stimulate inspiration. Because the diaphragm and intercostal muscles are skeletal, they will only contract when stimulated to do so by nerve impulses from motor neurones.

The two phrenic nerves leave the spinal cord via the cervical nerve roots 3, 4 and 5. (You may find the following rhyme helpful: 'C 3 4 5 keep the diaphragm alive'.) After passing through the chest, one phrenic nerve stimulates each side of the diaphragm. This explains why patients with high cervical spinal cord damage are unable to breathe. (Cervical vertebral damage must always be assumed in traumatized patients until X-rays can be taken.) Intercostal nerves leave the spinal cord via thoracic nerve roots to stimulate the intercostal muscles. When the inspiratory impulses generated in the medulla stop, the lungs and respiratory muscles passively recoil causing expiration.

The main additional factor stimulating respiration is increase in the levels of carbon dioxide in the blood. Increase in the plasma volumes of carbon dioxide is detected in the medulla, which then stimulates increased respiratory effort in order to excrete the excess.

Other factors that stimulate the respiratory centre include messages from chemoreceptors located in the aorta and carotid arteries. These specialized receptors detect falls in the level of oxygen; however, the degree to which oxygen lack stimulates respiration in normal physiology is small compared to the effect of carbon dioxide increase. Patients with chronic bronchitis have difficulty excreting carbon dioxide so their blood levels of this waste gas are chronically high; this overwhelms the carbon dioxide detectors in the respiratory centre of the medulla. The result of this is that excess carbon dioxide no longer stimulates the respiratory drive; as a result, such individuals become dependent on this secondary, oxygen-lack drive, from chemoreceptors. If these patients are given high concentrations of oxygen this may switch off their oxygen-lack respiratory drive, causing them to stop breathing. However, in people without chronic airways disease it is quite safe to give high concentrations of oxygen when required.

Respiration may be stimulated by messages from the higher centres of the brain, for example in anxiety. Decreased pH of the blood may also stimulate respiration; this is seen in the 'air hunger' characteristic of ketoacidosis in poorly managed diabetes.

Essential science

In order to understand internal respiration and many other aspects of physiology it is necessary to have some knowledge of elements, compounds and chemical reactions.

Elements

An element is a pure substance that cannot be chemically split into simpler substances. There are 95 naturally occurring elements, although people have made a few more using nuclear physics. All substances are made up of various proportions of these basic building blocks, chemically combined in various proportions. Symbols are used as shorthand to identify elements; the following selection shows some of those we frequently come across in physiology and nursing.

Hydrogen H	Carbon C	Nitrogen N	Oxygen O
Fluorine F	Sodium Na	Magnesium Mg	Phosphorus P
Sulphur S	Chlorine Cl	Potassium K	Calcium Ca
Iron Fe	Copper Cu	Zinc Zn	Selenium Se
Iodine I	Mercury Hg	Lead Pb	

Compounds

When two or more elements chemically combine together a compound is formed. Individual atoms of the original element are combined into a molecule of compound. Water is a compound of hydrogen and oxygen; carbon dioxide is a compound of carbon and oxygen; sugars are compounds of carbon, hydrogen and oxygen. Although oxygen is an element, in gaseous form two atoms of oxygen combine to form a single oxygen molecule – this is referred to as a diatomic molecule. In a chemical formula the symbol for the element and number of atoms in the molecule are given.

Chemical reactions

These occur when two or more elements or compounds chemically interact together, resulting in the formation of new compounds, or liberation of elements. Chemical equations are used to record the original reactants and products. Because matter cannot be created or destroyed, the number of atoms of each element must always be the same before and after the reaction has occurred. Chemical bonds hold elements together in new compounds. The creation of new chemical bonds required an input of energy. For example, energy from sunlight is required in photosynthesis to synthesize sugars from water and carbon dioxide. When these bonds are broken down in internal respiration this energy is released and may be used to do useful work.

Internal respiration

Internal respiration is a term that should be restricted to describing the events that occur inside mitochondria located in the cells. Oxygen is essential to all animals. Each living cell must have a constant supply of oxygen if it is to survive. The reason oxygen is required is that all cells must produce energy to fuel the processes of life. Life needs energy. In the mitochondria glucose and other fuels (correctly termed metabolic substrates) are combined with oxygen to produce energy. When fuel molecules such as glucose are oxidized, the chemical bonds that held the atoms together are broken, with the effect of releasing the energy that was stored in those bonds. This energy was ultimately derived from sunlight when the fuel molecule was produced in the process of photosynthesis. Internal respiration may be summarized as follows:

Glucose + oxygen → water + carbon dioxide + energy

As a chemical formula, it can be represented like this:

$C_6H_{12}O_6 + 6O_2$ → $6H_2O + 6CO_2$ + energy

In order to oxidize one molecule of glucose, six molecules of oxygen are required. In addition to the energy derived, six molecules of water and carbon dioxide are also produced. This explains that the carbon, in exhaled carbon dioxide, is derived from ingested carbohydrates. The six H_2O molecules are referred to as metabolic water. The energy derived from this reaction is initially used to generate ATP from ADP.

ATP and ADP

Energy production in internal respiration is common to all animals and most bacteria. The process is termed oxidative phosphorylation. Oxygen is used to facilitate phosphorylation. This means the addition of a single phosphate unit to an existing two-phosphate unit. ADP (adenosine diphosphate) is converted to ATP (adenosine triphosphate). The bond between the single phosphate unit and the ADP is energy rich, and therefore energy is required to unite the phosphate unit with the ADP. However, when the phosphate unit dissociates from the ATP, energy that may be used in living processes is liberated. This liberation of energy where it is required converts the ATP back to ADP. In other words, the ATP stores energy in a chemical form and transfers it from the mitochondria where it is produced to wherever it is required. ATP is sometimes referred to as the 'energy currency' of the cell. Energy generation may be summarized as follows:

ADP + P + energy → ATP

When this energy is subsequently used in energy-demanding cellular processes the process may be summarized as follows:

ATP → ADP + P + energy

Hypoxia

This refers to a shortage of oxygen at the level of the tissues. This may arise because of a lack of oxygen in the atmosphere or drowning. In addition, hypoxia may develop if the mechanisms of ventilation are deficient; this may occur in some forms of paralysis when the respiratory muscles do not function normally. Almost any form of lung disease may lead to hypoxia. If the blood is unable to transport oxygen hypoxia will also result.

CHAPTER 8

The digestive system

Introduction

The functions of the digestive system can be summarized as ingestion, digestion, absorption and elimination. Ingestion refers to taking food into the body, the process of eating. Ingested food molecules, however, are often large and insoluble; in order for them to be absorbed into the body they must first be broken down into smaller units. The process of converting large, ingested foodstuffs into a form that may be absorbed is termed digestion. After food has been digested, it must then be absorbed into the blood and lymphatic systems of the body before it can be utilized. The process whereby digested food is transferred from the lumen of the gut into the circulatory systems is called absorption. Not all ingested material is absorbed – some continues along the length of the gut and is eliminated as waste. Fibre is not broken down by any digestive processes and is eliminated in the same form in which it was eaten.

Structures of the digestive system

Essentially, the gastrointestinal (GI) tract or gut is a single tube that runs from the mouth to the anus. (The old-fashioned name for the GI tract is the alimentary canal.) The digestive system consists of the organs that compose the GI tract and the accessory organs of digestion. These accessory organs are not part of the tract but produce and secrete enzymes essential for the digestive process. Different sections of the GI tract have different properties and diameters of lumen, which allow for the specific functions necessary.

Diagram 8.1
The principal
sections of the
GI tract.

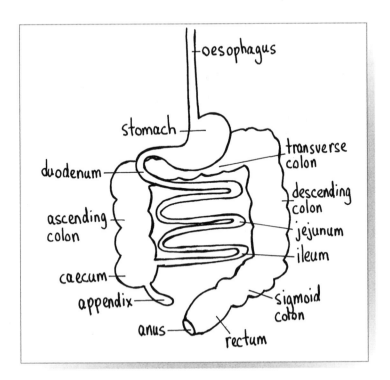

Diagram 8.1
The principal
sections of the
GI tract.

Layers

The walls of all the sections of the GI tract from the oesophagus to the rectum have the same basic layered structure. The lumen is surrounded by mucosa, submucosa, a muscular layer and an outer serosa.

Mucosa

The inner layer, immediately surrounding the lumen, is called the mucosa. This is composed of a mucous membrane lined with mucus. A mucous membrane is simply a layer of tissue that secretes mucus. Mucus protects the underlying cells and also acts as a lubricant to ease the passage of material along the lumen. The thickness of the mucosal epithelium varies along the length of the tract. In areas such as the mouth, oesophagus and anus, which are subject to a lot of mechanical forces and abrasion, the mucosa is composed of a stratified epithelium. In sections associated with absorption it is important for the lining to be thin to facilitate diffusion of nutrients. In these areas the mucosa is composed of a simple columnar epithelium.

Underneath the epithelium but still part of the mucosa is a layer of connective tissue containing small blood vessels. These vessels supply nutrients and oxygen to the epithelial cells. In some areas of the GI tract they may also be involved in the process of absorption. Under the connective tissue is a thin layer of smooth muscle. This supports the overlying connective and epithelial tissues and in some areas of the gut pulls the lining up into a series of folds. These folds have the effect of enlarging the internal surface area of the lumen thus increasing the rate of digestion and absorption.

Submucosa

The layer underneath the mucosa is called the submucosa. This is composed of loose connective tissue and also carries numerous blood vessels that perfuse the gut wall with blood. In certain areas of the GI tract, the submucosa contains exocrine glands that produce some of the digestive enzymes. Areas of lymphatic tissue are found in the submucosa; these are referred to as lymphatic nodules and provide an immune function. This layer also contains a network of intrinsic nerve fibres collectively called the submucosal plexus. ('Plexus' means 'a network of blood vessels or nerve fibres'.)

Muscular layer

Under the submucosa is the muscular layer or muscularis. There are two layers of smooth, involuntary muscle: the outer layer is composed of longitudinal muscle fibres and the inner layer of circular muscles. The wall of the stomach has an additional inner layer of muscle fibres, which run obliquely. Activity of the muscular layer is coordinated by a network of intrinsic, autonomic nerve fibres called the myenteric plexus.

Contraction and relaxation of these muscle layers allows material to be propelled along the GI tract. This muscular contraction also helps with the physical breakdown of food and aids the mixing in of digestive enzymes. In addition to the involuntary muscles found in the wall of the GI tract, the mouth, pharynx, oesophagus and anus also contain voluntary muscles.

Serosa

The outer layer of the gut wall is called the serosa. This is composed of loose connective tissue with a serous membrane on the external surface of the bowel. Like all serous membranes it secretes a small volume of serous fluid (fluid derived from serum, i.e. plasma) that acts as an external lubricant. Below the diaphragm, the serosal layer is called the visceral peritoneum.

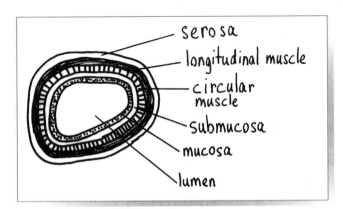

Diagram 8.2
Layers of the GI tract.

Peritoneum

This is the membrane that lines the surface of the organs in the abdominal cavity and also lines the inner abdominal wall. The peritoneum immediately surrounding the organs is referred to as visceral, and the layer lining the abdominal wall as parietal. Between these two layers is a potential space containing serous lubricating fluid. This allows areas of the intestine to move slightly relative to other lengths. The parietal peritoneal membrane contains many pain receptors, which make it a very sensitive tissue.

Sometimes as a result of infection, or after surgery, areas of the visceral and parietal peritoneum are physically connected by scar tissue; this disorder is referred to as adhesions, and it often requires surgery to separate them. If gastrointestinal contents escape through a perforation in the wall of the gut this will cause inflammation of the peritoneum, a life-threatening condition called peritonitis. In peritoneal dialysis, dialysing fluid is introduced between the parietal and visceral layers.

Mesentery

This is a double layer of peritoneum that connects the jejunum and ileum to the posterior abdominal wall. Blood vessels that supply the small intestine run between the layers of the mesentery, carrying blood from large blood vessels to the gut wall. Venous and lymphatic drainage vessels are also located in the mesentery. This arrangement keeps all of the vessels which supply and drain the intestines neatly in one place; if there were free individual vessels supplying areas of gut they could readily get tangled up.

The mesentery is fan shaped, starting with a 15 cm length that connects the whole structure to the posterior body wall; this is called the root of the mesentery. By the time the same double sheet of mesentery reaches the small intestine it is 6 metres long. Despite this length, the height is only 20 cm at the centre and much less towards the edges. Major blood vessels supplying the gut run behind the peritoneum, so branches of the aorta project through the root of the mesentery, and travel through the mesentery to the small intestine. In the same way venous branches drain from the gut, through the mesentery, then through the root of the mesentery into branches of what will become the hepatic portal vein.

There is a similar double layer of tissue called the mesocolon that connects the duodenum and part of the colon to the posterior abdominal wall.

Three main blood vessels supply the GI tract. The coeliac artery leaves the aorta and divides to perfuse the stomach, duodenum, liver and spleen. Blood is supplied to the rest of the small intestine via the superior mesenteric artery, which also supplies the ascending and most of the transverse colon. Remaining areas of the colon are supplied by the inferior mesenteric artery. Venous drainage occurs via splenic and gastric veins with an inferior and superior mesenteric vein, all of which drain directly into the hepatic portal vein to convey blood to the liver.

Omentum

The greater omentum is a large, apron-like fold of tissue that lies in front of the organs of the GI tract. This structure stores adipose tissue and is one reason why people often get a fat stomach when they become obese.

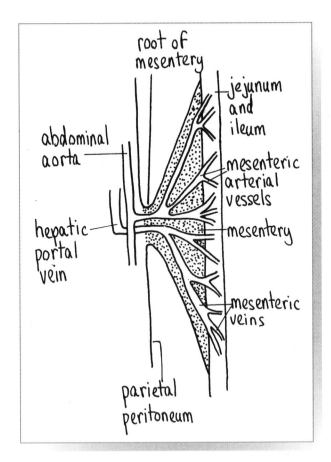

root of
mesentery

jejunum
and
ileum

abdominal
aorta

mesenteric
arterial
vessels

mesentery

hepatic
portal
vein

mesenteric
veins

parietal
peritoneum

Diagram 8.3 Blood vessels to and from most of the small intestines run in between the layers of the mesentery. Starting from a 15 cm connection, the mesentery provides vascular and neuronal support for a 6 metre length of small intestine. For simplicity this diagram shows the arterial supply at the top and the venous drainage at the bottom. In reality, arterial, venous, lymphatic and nervous connections run together.

However, the omentum is also called the 'policeman of the abdomen'. This is because it is able to seal off and consolidate areas of infection, which prevents spread throughout the peritoneal cavity. Infection in the peritoneal cavity is called peritonitis and is life-threatening.

Principles of regulation

The activity of the GI tract and accessory organs must be controlled and regulated. This is achieved by neural and hormonal control mechanisms. There are two aspects to neural control, referred to as intrinsic and extrinsic. The intrinsic nerves are autonomic fibres located in the walls of the tract that coordinate local muscular and secretory activity. Extrinsic nervous control involves autonomic nerves that communicate directly with the central nervous system. Afferent, sensory neurons convey information from the gut into the CNS. Efferent, motor fibres carry information from the CNS to coordinate the activity of the digestive system. There are some sympathetic fibres involved in control of the gut but most of the extrinsic neuronal control is parasympathetic, often via the vagus nerve.

Some of the cells that line the gut produce endocrine hormones. These specialized cells are called enteroendocrine cells. The hormones they produce are systemically absorbed but affect and regulate other organs of the digestive system.

Appetite

The desire to eat is stimulated by a specialized group of neurones in the hypothalamus that form the appetite centre. It is the hypothalamus that generates the sensation of hunger and the desire to search for food. In addition, eating increases the release of dopamine from some areas of the brain, which generates a sensation of pleasure. If a person has experienced pleasure in the past from eating a particular food they will have a desire to reproduce this sensation by further eating. When enough food has been eaten another area of the hypothalamus produces a feeling of satisfaction. This group of neurones is referred to as the satiety centre.

Peristalsis

This is the term used to describe the coordinated waves of muscular contraction that occur in the walls of the gut. Muscles in a short length of the GI tract will contract, while those immediately in front relax. This allows contents to be squeezed along a length of lumen. The area of muscle that was relaxed then contracts, while the length in front of this section will relax, propelling the material further forward. The result is that waves of contraction pass along the length of the gut wall, progressively transferring material from mouth to anus. Peristalsis should always occur in the mouth to anus direction; in vomiting, however, material is propelled in the opposite direction by antiperistalsis in the wall of the oesophagus.

Diagram 8.4 A food bolus is propelled along a length of GI tract by a wave of peristalsis. Arrows indicate the direction of bolus movement.

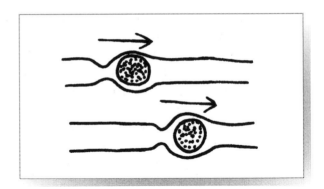

Digestion

In digestion, food molecules are broken down into simpler components that may later be absorbed. Proteins are broken down into amino acids, carbohydrates into simple sugars, and fats into fatty acids and glycerol. There are two ways this is achieved, mechanical and chemical.

Mechanical

Food is physically broken down by chewing (or mastication) in the mouth. Once food is in the stomach there are regular peristaltic contractions about every 20 seconds, called mixing waves. These churn the gastric contents into a mixture called chyme. There are further mechanical effects as chyme is peristaltically squeezed along the small intestine.

Digestive enzymes and enzyme precursors

In Chapter 1 we considered intracellular enzymes, which catalysed all biochemical reactions in the cell. The enzymes concerned with digestion, however, only break down large molecules into smaller ones. Digestive enzymes are produced by exocrine glands and act in the lumen of the gut.

Many digestive enzymes are made as enzyme precursors to prevent the enzyme products digesting the glands in which they are produced. Enzyme precursors are normally converted into an active form of enzyme in the lumen of the GI tract. For example, trypsin is an enzyme which will digest proteins; this is formed as trypsinogen in the pancreas. Trypsinogen is inactive and will not break down protein molecules. However, when exported from the pancreas into the lumen of the small intestine, it is then converted into an active form. If it were synthesized as end-produce trypsin in the pancreas, the pancreas would itself be digested as it is largely composed of protein. Active enzymes are unable to damage body tissues in the gut lumen as the mucosa is protected by a layer of mucus.

Mouth

Teeth

Children have 20 deciduous or 'milk' teeth. Adults should have 32 teeth, shaped to perform particular functions. The incisors at the front are chisel-shaped to bite into food, for example, cutting into an apple. Behind these are the canines, which are pointed to stab into and tear food, such as tearing off a piece of meat. Next there are the premolars; these crush and grind food so are important in eating vegetables and grains. Finally, at the back of the mouth are the molars which also crush and grind. The upper and lower jawbones each have two pairs of incisors, one pair of canines, two pairs of premolars and three pairs of molars.

Teeth are lined with hard enamel; under this is a bone-like substance called dentine. The inner pulp cavity contains nerves, blood and lymphatic vessels. Cementum holds teeth into the jawbone.

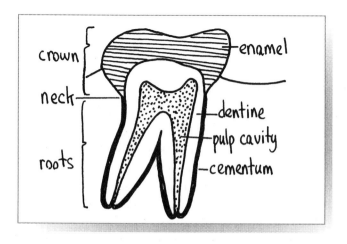

Diagram 8.5
Generalized structure of a tooth.

Saliva

Three pairs of salivary glands produce saliva, which is drained into the mouth via salivary ducts. Saliva is continually secreted in small volumes to keep the mouth moist; however, the sight, smell or taste of food may increase production by as much as 20 times. Secretion of saliva is stimulated by activity of the parasympathetic nervous system under the control of two salivary nuclei located in the brain stem. Water is the principal component of saliva but it also contains some sodium chloride and an enzyme that acts against bacteria called lysozyme. Mucus acts as a lubricant and softening agent. Salivary amylase is the digestive enzyme present, and starts the digestion of carbohydrates by breaking starch molecules into maltose. Starch is a polysaccharide; this means it is composed of a long chain of sugar units chemically bonded together. A single sugar unit is referred to as a monosaccharide, while a two-sugar unit is a disaccharide. Amylase breaks some of the bonds holding the individual sugar units together, resulting in maltose – a disaccharide.

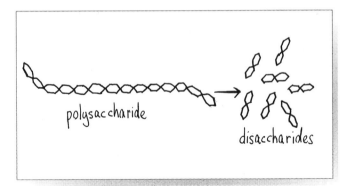

Diagram 8.6
Amylase breaks polysaccharide chains down into disaccharides.

Eating and swallowing

The teeth close on food, which is thereby crushed and displaced. The tongue, lips and cheeks repeatedly push the food back between the teeth for further mechanical processing. During this grinding process, food is mixed with saliva and formed into a bolus.

Swallowing (or deglutition) occurs in stages. First, the mouth is closed. Next, starting from the front, the tongue moves the food backwards along the palate, which forms the roof of the mouth, towards the oropharynx. Contact of the food bolus with the back of the mouth initiates the swallowing reflex. Respiration is stopped as part of the reflex to prevent aspiration of food into the trachea.

Return of food back into the mouth is prevented by the tongue, and food is also prevented from going up into the nose. Movement of the epiglottis prevents food entering the trachea. Next, the muscular walls of the pharynx contract, pushing the food in the only direction left open, into the oesophagus.

Oesophagus

This is a muscular tube that extends from the laryngopharynx down through the chest. It passes through the diaphragm into the abdominal cavity where it joins the stomach. Oesophageal lumen is lined with stratified squamous epithelium; mucus is secreted from this lining to lubricate the passage of food.

At the bottom end of the oesophagus the cardiac sphincter prevents reflux of gastric contents. If acid contents from the stomach do reflux into the oesophagus 'heartburn' is usually experienced. Once a food bolus enters the oesophagus, peristaltic waves of contraction in the muscular wall propel food down to the stomach. As a food bolus nears the cardiac sphincter the muscles in this area relax to allow the food to pass into the stomach. Evidence for the peristaltic action of the oesophagus is seen in the ability to swallow when upside-down.

Difficulty in swallowing is called dysphagia; it may be caused by diseases of the mouth or tongue, neuromuscular disorders, oesophageal disorders, foreign bodies or psychological problems. If food enters the airway when an individual is conscious this will lead to choking; the most common cause of this is trying to talk and eat at the same time. As unconscious patients are unable to swallow they must never be given anything by mouth; it will simply run down into the lungs, causing aspiration of the food or fluid.

Stomach

Basic structure

The stomach is a widened area of the GI tract that expands when it fills with food. It receives, stores and mechanically and chemically breaks down food. Finally, it controls the release of gastric contents into the first stage of the small intestine ('gastric' simply means 'to do with the stomach'). This gastric emptying is regulated via a second ring of muscle called the pyloric sphincter.

The proximal (first part) of the stomach has a relatively thin wall and is highly distendable, allowing it to store an ingested meal. The distal (lower) part of the stomach has a thicker muscular layer and has a greater level of peristaltic activity to churn the contents. Anatomically, the upper area of the stomach is called the fundus, the middle area the body and the lower area the pylorus.

Diagram 8.7

Areas and sphincters associated with the stomach.

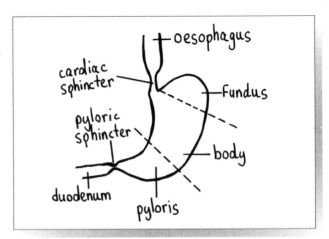

Mucosa of the stomach

Gastric mucosa lies in large folds called rugae when the stomach is empty. These increase the surface area of the stomach and allow for expansion after meals. Gastric lumen is lined with simple columnar epithelial cells. Close inspection of the mucosa lining reveals numerous gastric pits that project down into the mucosa. These pits contain the gastric glands.

Gastric glands are lined with several types of specialized exocrine cells that secrete the various gastric juices. Around the necks of the pits are mucous cells that secrete mucus. This is essential to protect the stomach lining from the irritating effect of other gastric juices. If the mucous lining is disrupted a gastric ulcer may result as gastric juices attack and digest underlying tissue.

The chief cells (also called zymogenic cells) are the most common cell type in the pits. These produce the enzyme precursor called pepsinogen; this travels out of the gastric pit into the lumen of the stomach. Parietal cells (also called oxyntic cells) secrete hydrochloric acid. This is a very strong acid that kills most potential pathogens that might be ingested. Intrinsic factor is also secreted by the parietal cells; this is a glycoprotein that binds with vitamin B12 to allow this nutrient to be later absorbed in the small intestine. Without intrinsic factor this vitamin cannot be absorbed and pernicious anaemia will result. Gastric juice is a combination of these secretory products in a watery medium.

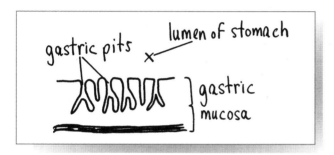

Diagram 8.8
Gastric mucosa with pits containing gastric glands.

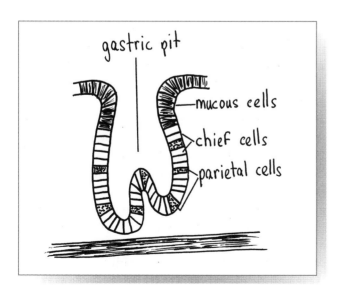

Diagram 8.9 A gastric pit, at higher magnification. Gastric glands, which secrete gastric juice, are formed as gastric pits in the mucosa.

Gastric regulation

Nerve signals from the parasympathetic vagus nerve increase the secretion of gastric juice. In addition to this neuronal control, the presence of proteins in the stomach initiates secretion of gastrin from specialized mucosal cells. Gastrin is an endocrine hormone that circulates in the blood and stimulates the chief cells to secrete more pepsinogen and the parietal cells to produce more hydrochloric acid. Protein in the stomach therefore stimulates the secretion of the digestive agents necessary for its own digestion. When there is no protein in the stomach the levels of pepsin and hydrochloric acid are comparatively low. This mechanism reduces the volumes of gastric juice when the stomach is empty so helps to protect the lining from the potential harmful effects of pepsin and hydrochloric acid.

Histamine is also produced by gastric mucosa. Parietal cells are able to detect this chemical via histamine type 2 (H_2) receptors. Histamine stimulates the parietal cells to secrete more hydrochloric acid. Drugs such as cimetidine and ranitidine reduce gastric acid by blocking the H_2 receptor sites on the parietal cells. This reduction in gastric acid can aid in the healing of peptic ulcers.

Chemical digestion in the stomach

Once in the lumen of the stomach pepsinogen is converted into the active proteolytic enzyme called pepsin. 'Lytic' or 'lysis' means 'to break down', so a proteolytic enzyme will break down proteins. A protein is made up of a long chain of individual amino acid units joined together by peptide bonds. Pepsin starts the process of protein digestion by breaking some of the peptide bonds, which results in shorter lengths of amino acid sequences called peptides.

Normally the names of all enzymes end with the suffix '-ase'; however, pepsin was discovered before this convention was adopted. In young children the stomach also secretes rennin; this coagulates milk into a curd to prevent it running through the stomach before it has time to be acted on by pepsin.

Once chemical digestion has occurred, the combination of gastric peristalsis and relaxation of the pyloric sphincter will move partly digested chyme into the small intestine. Chyme is the name given to the combination of partly digested food mixed with digestive juices. The rate of gastric emptying varies from 2 to 6 hours depending on the

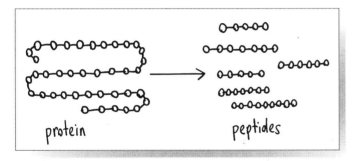

protein   peptides

Diagram 8.10 Proteins are
long chains of amino acid.
Pepsin breaks these sequences
down into smaller peptides.

nature of the food contained. Carbohydrates pass through the stomach
fairly quickly but foods containing proteins take longer. Emptying is
slowest after meals that contain a lot of fat. The rate of stomach emptying is limited by the rates at which the small intestine can process
particular food types.

Absorption from the stomach

There is some absorption from the stomach into the blood. This is
clearly limited by the large size of the undigested and partly digested
food molecules; however, water and alcohol will be absorbed, as they
are already small soluble molecules.

Liver and pancreas

These accessory organs of the digestive system produce juices and
enzymes essential to the digestive process. The liver produces bile.
Although this is essentially an excretory product, largely derived from
the destruction of old red blood cells, it also plays an active role in
digestion. Bile from the liver passes out via the right and left hepatic
ducts, which unite to form the common hepatic duct. Freshly formed
bile then travels along the cystic duct into the gall bladder where it is
stored and concentrated. When required, the gall bladder contracts

and bile passes down the common bile duct. The common bile duct joins with the pancreatic duct forming a common duct called the ampulla of the bile duct; this structure then communicates with the lumen of the duodenum. Reflux from the duodenum into the ampulla is prevented by the sphincter of Oddi.

In addition to the endocrine functions of the pancreas (discussed in Chapter 3) it also produces digestive enzymes. The exocrine secretory regions produce enzymes which drain via small pancreatic ducts into a large pancreatic duct, which in turn leaves the gland to join the common bile duct at the ampulla. There is also a smaller accessory pancreatic duct that enters the duodenum separately. Pancreatic juice contains pancreatic amylase, pancreatic lipase, chymotrypsinogen and trypsinogen. Sodium bicarbonate is also produced, which gives pancreatic juice an alkaline pH.

Regulation of the liver and pancreas

The arrival of chyme in the duodenum and upper parts of the jejunum stimulates the release of an endocrine hormone called cholecystokinin (CCK). This is produced by specialized cells in the duodenal mucosa. As an endocrine hormone, CCK circulates in the blood and stimulates the secretion of pancreatic digestive enzymes. It also causes contraction of the gallbladder, which leads to bile passing down the common bile duct into the duodenum. As in the stomach, it is the arrival of food that stimulates the release of the agents required for digestion of that food.

Small intestine

The small intestine is a muscular tube about 6 metres long. It is arranged in three segments: the first is the duodenum which is only about 25 cm long; the second segment is the jejunum which is about 2.5 metres in length. The final 3.5 metre section is the ileum.

Chyme leaving the stomach trickles into the duodenum. About halfway along the duodenum a duct enters from the ampulla of the pancreatic and biliary systems. Bile is not a digestive enzyme; its role is to emulsify fats into small globules. This emulsification greatly increases the surface area of fat and therefore the speed of its digestion when it is subsequently exposed to juices from the pancreas. (Milk is an example of a fat emulsion.)

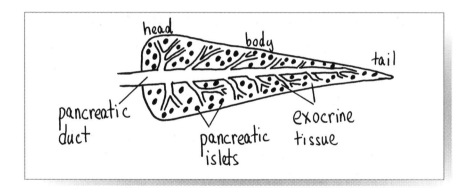

Diagram 8.11
The pancreas is described
as an organ with a head,
body and tail.

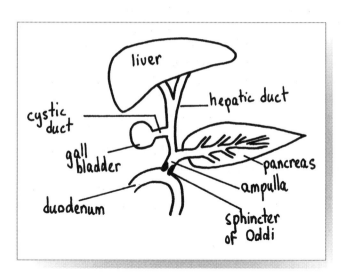

Diagram 8.12 The liver,
biliary system, pancreas
and ducts.

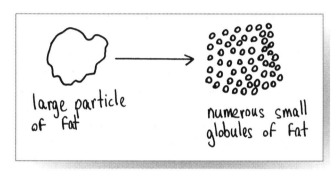

Diagram 8.13
Fat before and after
emulsification by bile.

Chemical digestion in the small intestine

There are two sources of digestive enzymes active in the small intestine. First, enzymes are produced in the pancreas. Second, enzymes derive from cells that line much of the internal surface of the small intestine. These specialized lining cells are called enterocytes. As nutrients are absorbed and pass through these epithelial cells further digestion occurs. Enzymes located in the enterocytes include the carbohydrate-digesting enzymes – maltase, sucrase and lactase – and a few protein-digesting enzymes referred to as peptidases.

Proteins

Pancreatic juice enters the duodenum through the same duct as the bile. In the lumen of the bowel, inactive trypsinogen is converted into trypsin by the action of enterokinase, an enzyme secreted by the mucosa of the small intestine. Once activated, trypsin in turn activates chymotrypsinogen into chymotrypsin. This arrangement prevents conversion of proteolytic enzyme precursors into their active form before they reach the mucus-protected gut lumen. Trypsin and chymotrypsin then both act to break down lengths of proteins and peptides into smaller peptide units. The three protein-digesting enzymes mentioned so far – pepsin, trypsin and chymotrypsin – are all required to break down proteins because individually they break the peptide bonds between different amino acids. The final phase of protein breakdown occurs mostly in and near the enterocytes. Peptidases from the enterocytes complete the breakdown of peptides into individual amino acids.

Carbohydrates

Some carbohydrate is broken down by salivary amylase; however, its action is blocked by the acid environment of the stomach. Pancreatic amylase continues the breakdown of starch, a polysaccharide, into disaccharide sugars. Disaccharides are molecules made up of two monosaccharide units. The final digestion of these disaccharide sugars is completed by the carbohydrate-digesting enzymes of the enterocytes. These contain maltase which breaks down maltose into two molecules of glucose. Lactase breaks down the milk sugar lactose into one molecule of glucose and one of galactose. Sucrase breaks down sucrose into one molecule of glucose and one of fructose. This means the end product of all carbohydrate digestion is monosaccharide single-unit sugars.

Lipids

Lipid is another name for fats. Fats are first emulsified into very small globules by bile. Pancreatic lipase then breaks down lipid molecules into their component parts, which are fatty acids and glycerol.

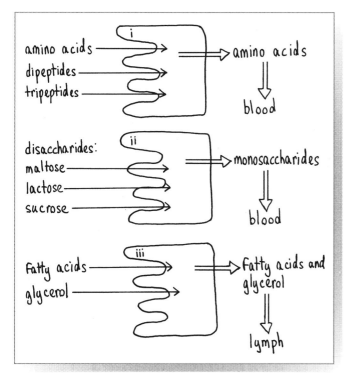

Diagram 8.14 The final phase of digestion occurs as nutrients pass through enterocytes. In reality a single enterocyte contains a range of enzymes but these are illustrated one at a time.
(i) Action of peptidases.
(ii) Action of maltase, lactase and sucrase.
(iii) Absorption of the products of fat digestion.

Intestinal juice

Between the individual villi are small pits called crypts of Lieberkuhn. These crypts are lined with a few goblet cells for the production of mucus. In addition, there is a large number of enterocytes that secrete large quantities of water and electrolytes. These secretions, called intestinal juice, do not contain digestive enzymes but wash out of the crypt over the surface of the villi. This provides a watery medium for the absorption of the products of digestion from the lumen into the enterocytes of the villi.

Absorption

Around 90% of absorption takes place in the small intestine, primarily in the jejunum and ileum. The remaining 10% of absorption from the gut takes place from the stomach and colon. In order for absorption to be efficient, a large surface area is required into which the products of digestion can enter. The lining of the small intestine has circular folds. These project areas of mucosa into the lumen to increase surface area. The folds extend from about half to two thirds of the way around the lumen and are up to 8 mm deep.

In addition, the circular folds themselves have a highly infolded surface, being covered with villi. These small projections, 0.5–1 mm high, further increase the surface area. Villi are lined with epithelial cells called enterocytes, the surface of which is also highly infolded. Numerous small projections termed microvilli project from the surface of the enterocytes. Each individual cell has about 3 000 microvilli. Collectively the microvilli form a striated or brush border about 1 μm micrometre thick. These three levels of infolding massively increase the surface area for absorption, and so for the final digestion of food in the enterocytes.

Villi contain a central lymphatic vessel called a lacteal. Most fatty acids and glycerol absorb into the lacteal and are drained into the central lymphatic system. From here, they travel with the lymphatic fluid and eventually enter the blood via the left lymphatic duct, which drains into the subclavian vein. An arteriole feeds blood into each individual villus; this breaks into a capillary network that is subsequently drained into a venule. All of the products of digestion that are not absorbed into the lymphatic lacteal pass into the capillary blood of the villi. Veins draining the intestine combine to form the hepatic portal vein which carries blood directly to the liver, as discussed in Chapter 4.

Essential science

Fat and water solubility

It is a common observation that fat and water do not mix. If I pour some cooking oil on to water, it forms globules of fat. This occurs because the fat molecules will stick together and at the same time repel water molecules. If I then add a water-soluble molecule such as sugar, this will dissolve into the water but not into the fat. In the same way, if I add a fat-soluble molecule such as vitamin A, this will dissolve into the oil but not into the water. Fat-soluble molecules are described as being lipophilic: 'lipo-' relates to fat and '-philic' means love, so these are literally 'fat-loving' molecules. At the same time as being lipophilic, most fat-soluble molecules are also hydrophobic: 'hydro-' means water and '-phobic' relates to fear; literally this means 'water-fearing'. In practice, this means fat-soluble molecules repel water.

This is an important principle in physiology and pharmacology as only molecules with a fat-soluble component will diffuse through cell membranes, which are mostly composed of lipids. Fatty cell membranes have hydrophobic properties so tend to repel water-soluble molecules.

Mechanisms of absorption

There are two mechanisms used to transfer the products of digestion from the gut lumen into the blood or lymphatic systems. The first is simple diffusion. Because the epithelium of the small intestine is thin, soluble molecules will diffuse from an area of high concentration to one of low concentration. This mechanism is, however, dependent on the nutrient molecule being able to diffuse across the cell membranes of the cells that line the gut lumen. As cell membranes are largely composed of lipids, only small or fat-soluble molecules may freely diffuse across. Fatty acids and glycerol are therefore able to be absorbed by diffusion. Most of the small molecules such as water, minerals and vitamins also simply diffuse into the villi.

As amino acids and sugars are water-soluble they do not diffuse through the lipid-based enterocyte cell membranes effectively. This means these molecules must be specially transported if they are to be absorbed efficiently. This second process is called active transport. 'Active' implies the use of energy, so this process uses ATP as an energy source to facilitate the movement. Enterocyte cell membranes contain specialized transmembrane proteins which act as a 'gate' into the cell, through which sugars and amino acids may pass. Because this process is active it may work against the prevailing diffusion gradient.

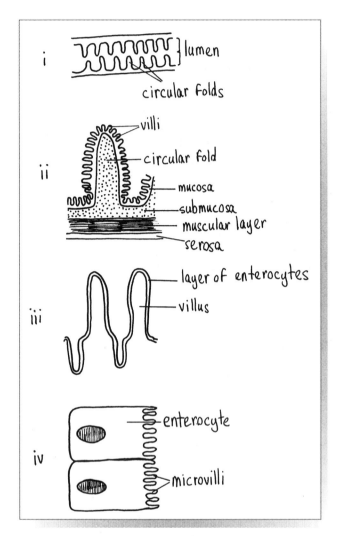

Diagram 8.15 These four diagrams represent progressively increasing powers of magnification. Three levels of infolding massively increase the internal surface area of the intestine.

(i) Circular folds project into the lumen of the intestine.

(ii) Villi cover the circular folds.

(iii) An individual villi is lined with enterocytes.

(iv) Enterocyte surface area is increased by numerous microvilli.

Secretion and reabsorption

The GI tract secretes large volumes of fluids into the lumen to facilitate the processes of digestion and absorption. In addition to the fluid we drink, every day we swallow about 1 litre of saliva. Gastric secretions add 1.5 litres of fluid and bile about a further 1 litre. Total volumes of intestinal juice are around 2 litres per day. Even the colon secretes approximately 200 ml of fluid over a 24-hour period. The majority of these fluids are reabsorbed by the small intestine, although significant volumes must be reabsorbed from the colon.

Diagram 8.16
Absorption of nutrients into the villi. Fatty acids and glycerol enter the lymphatic lacteal, water-soluble nutrients enter the capillaries.

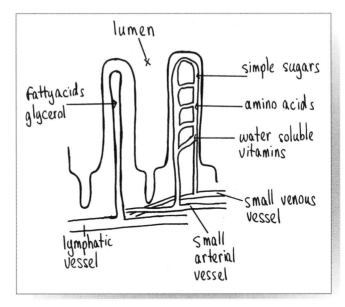

Diagram 8.17 Example of an active transport system. A water-soluble nutrient enters the start of the transmembrane gate. Using energy derived from ATP, the protein then alters position to transport the nutrient through the cell membrane. After this the same protein will swing back again, ready to transport the next nutrient molecule. (This is also a good example of the importance of protein molecules being arranged into a particular shape.)

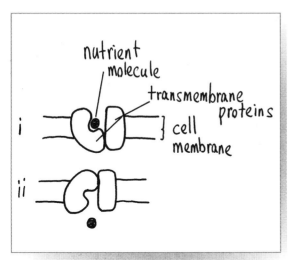

Colon

Components

Fairly large volumes of watery chyme enter the colon (or large intestine) from the ileum, via the ileocaecal valve. Anatomically, the colon is divided into several sections. The first part is the caecum; the appendix is a blind-ended projection of this structure. Next, the ascending colon rises up the right side of the abdomen to the area of the liver; here it bends to the left at the hepatic flexure. 'Flexure' just means bend, so this is the 'bend near the liver'. The transverse colon runs from right to left, near the top of the abdomen, before turning down near the spleen at the bend called the splenic flexure. The descending colon runs down the left side of the abdominal cavity and extends into the sigmoid colon, which passes back in the direction of the anus. The rectum is between the sigmoid colon and the anus. The anus is a sphincter of muscle that regulates the exit of faeces from the rectum.

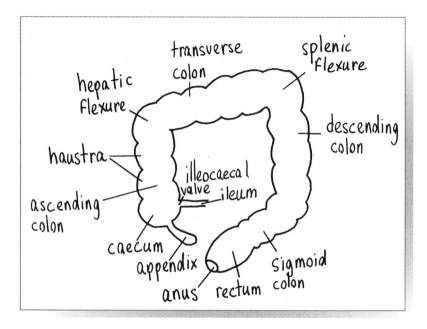

Diagram 8.18
Sections of the colon.

Absorption from the colon

The colon absorbs a lot of water from the chyme. This is important to prevent excessive water loss from the body. As well as preventing an inconvenient, near constant flow of watery faecal material from the anus, reabsorption is essential to prevent dehydration. Material that remains after the water has been absorbed becomes semi-solid faeces. Absorption of water from the colon is mostly by the passive process of osmosis. Water-soluble vitamins and electrolytes such as sodium and potassium are also absorbed from the colon.

There are a large number of bacteria living in the colon; these produce vitamin K, which is also locally absorbed. Bacteria in the colon comprise the normal 'flora' of the large intestine and prevent colonization with potentially pathogenic bacteria or fungi. This is why antibiotics may cause diarrhoea. Systemic antibiotics kill many of the bacteria and so disturb the natural balance between the flora and the colon.

Motility

Rates of peristalsis in the colon are generally slower than in the stomach and small intestine. The colon is arranged in a series of 'pouches' called haustra. As an individual pouch or haustrum is filling up it will relax to allow distension. However, once the wall is stretched to a particular point, contraction will be stimulated which passes the contents along to the next pouch or haustrum. In addition to this low-grade level of activity, from time to time there is a dramatic increase in the rate of peristalsis. This occurs from about the middle of the transverse colon into the descending colon. In some people, this mass peristalsis is stimulated by eating, the so-called gastrocolonic reflex. In others, it occurs at a particular time of day. This mass movement has the effect of moving the now faecal material down into the rectum. When material arrives in the rectum, this stretches the rectal walls, which brings about the desire to defecate.

In defecation the sphincter of the anus relaxes while the walls of the rectum contract. This muscular contraction tends to increase the pressure in the rectum, causing the faeces to be expelled through the anus. Further pressure is exerted on the rectum by the downward movement of the diaphragm and contraction of the muscles of the abdominal wall. Pressure on the rectum is further increased if the person is in a squatting position. This is one reason patients find it difficult to defecate into a bedpan if they are lying flat.

Diarrhoea

Inflammation of the lining of the intestine may be caused by infection with viruses, bacteria or protozoa. The natural response of the gut to such an infection is to secrete more intestinal fluids and increase the motility of the bowel. Large volumes of secreted fluid will physically flush disease-causing organisms along the lumen of the gut. Increased motility will hurry the infection through, before it has time to increase in severity. Watery flowing stools will therefore act as a natural cleansing mechanism, flushing large numbers of bacteria or viruses out of the body. This is why drugs to prevent diarrhoea are usually a bad idea; however, fluids and electrolytes should be replaced by eating and drinking. This replacement therapy is especially important in children, who have small volumes of body water and may rapidly become dehydrated.

CHAPTER 9

The urinary system

Components

The urinary system consists of the organs and structures which pro-duce, transport and store urine. Urine is produced in the kidneys and is transported to the urinary bladder by the right and left ureter. From time to time the bladder is emptied and urine is voided from the body via the urethra.

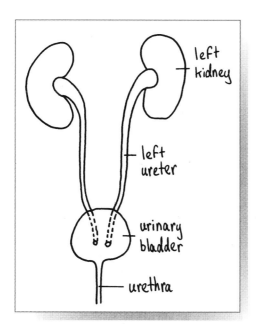

Diagram 9.1
Components of the urinary system.

The kidneys

Metabolic processes are carried out by all living cells. As a result of this biochemical activity, waste products are produced. If these are allowed to build up in body fluids, they will soon reach toxic levels. The kidneys are able to isolate and concentrate waste products in urine, which are then excreted from the body.

There are two kidneys located high in the abdominal cavity, on the posterior abdominal wall. Kidneys are dark red, bean-shaped organs. The right kidney is a little lower than the left due to the presence of the liver above. Because of the domed nature of the diaphragm the upper part of the kidneys receive some protection from the lower ribs. In addition the kidneys are embedded in a protective layer of perirenal fat ('renal' means 'to do with the kidneys').

Macroscopic structure

Surrounding the outer surface of each kidney is a layer of collagen-rich fibrous tissue that comprises the renal capsule.

The outer layer of the kidney itself is called the cortex. Under the cortex is a layer referred to as the medulla. The renal medulla is composed of structures called renal pyramids. The number of renal pyramids varies between individuals; there are normally between five and eleven per kidney. Between the renal pyramids of the medulla are projections from the cortex referred to as renal columns. The inner area of the kidney is called the renal pelvis, which is continuous with the ureter.

An arrangement of minor and major calyces connect the renal medulla with the renal pelvis. Calyces are essentially branches of the renal pelvis. Minor calyces form around the apex of the pyramids of the medulla and merge into larger calyces which then expand to form the pelvis.

At the centre of the concave side of the kidney is the region called the renal hilum. A hilum is a relatively small area where blood vessels, nerves and lymphatic vessels enter and leave an organ. The inner surface of the hilum is called the renal sinus, a hollow area within the kidney that contains the renal pelvis. It is via the hilum that the arteries, veins, lymphatics, nerves and ureters enter and leave each kidney. There are two adrenal glands, located one on top of each kidney (this is why these structures used to be called the suprarenal glands).

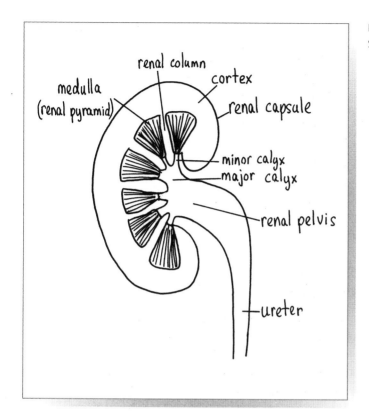

Diagram 9.2
Structure of a kidney.

Blood supply

Blood is transported to each kidney via a short branch from the aorta called the renal artery. The renal artery rapidly divides into segmental arteries, each perfusing a segment of the kidney. There are further rapid divisions of the branches of the renal artery until it breaks down into arterioles that are described as afferent. After blood has passed through the kidney, it is collected by a number of venous branches that unite to form a single renal vein. This vessel then returns blood directly to the inferior vena cava.

The kidneys have a large blood supply in relation to their size. Despite only comprising around 0.5% of body mass, in an average 70 kg adult the kidneys receive about 1200 mls of blood per minute. This is about 20% of total cardiac output at rest. Blood draining from the renal veins is not fully deoxygenated, indicating kidneys receive more blood than is required for purposes of oxygenation.

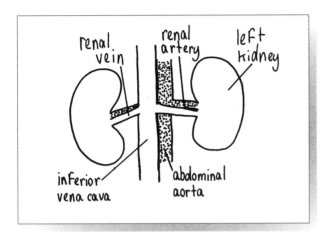

Diagram 9.3 Blood supply to and from the kidneys.

The nephrons

These are the functional renal units; there are about one million in each kidney. Each nephron consists of a renal tubule and an associated vascular system. The start of the tubule is a structure called the glomerular (Bowman's) capsule; this is located in the cortex of the kidney. Squamous cells comprise an outer or parietal layer of this capsule, while the inner or visceral layer is made up of specialized cells called podocytes. Between the two layers is a capsular space. Each nephron is supplied with blood from an afferent arteriole that opens into a ball of capillaries called the glomerulus. Glomerular capillaries are located inside the glomerular capsule. The combination of the glomerulus and the glomerular capsule is referred to as a renal corpuscle.

The glomerular capsule is continuous with the next section of the renal tubule called the first or proximal convoluted tubule. 'Convoluted' means 'coiled'; the result of this coiling is that a greater length of tubule can be contained in a smaller area. From here the tubule forms a loop; often this is a long loop dipping right down into the medulla of the kidney, which is called the loop of the nephron (or loop of Henle). This rises again, back towards the cortex, where it is formed into a second or distal convoluted tubule before connecting to a collecting duct.

Once blood has passed through the capillaries of the glomerulus it is drained via a second, efferent arteriole. This second arteriole then breaks up into a second capillary bed, which wraps itself around the renal tubule.

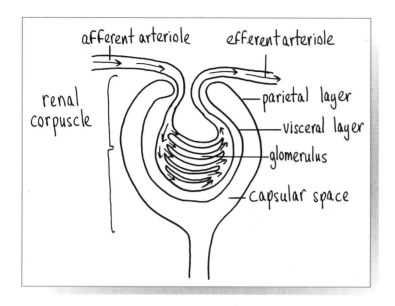

Diagram 9.4 A glomerular capsule and the glomerulus. The glomerulus is actually a sphere of capillaries. Arrows indicate direction of blood flow.

Formation of urine

Endothelial-capsular membrane

Endothelial cells of the glomerular capillaries contain pores that are too small to allow blood cells to pass through. However, smaller components of the blood may pass out of the capillaries via these small spaces. The basement membrane of the capillaries is on the outside of the cells that comprise the capillary wall. This membrane acts a further filter, preventing the escape of plasma proteins. Surrounding the endothelial cells of the capillaries of the glomerulus and their basement membrane are the podocytes.

Podocytes form the inner or visceral layer of the glomerular capsule. These cells have fine extensions called pedicels that wrap around the glomerular capillaries and form a physical sieve. The areas between the pedicels are called filtration slits.

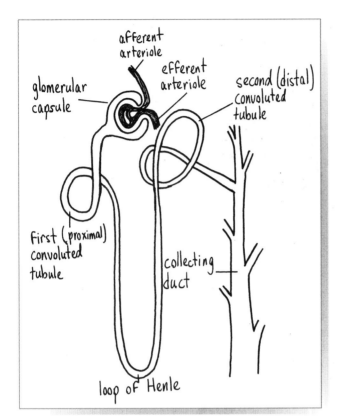

Diagram 9.5 Components of a renal tubule or nephron. The branched nature of the collecting duct indicates where other nephrons drain into the same duct.

Collectively the endothelium of the capillaries, the basement membrane and the podocytes form the endothelial-capsular membrane. This is the dialysing membrane of the kidney. Dialysis is a physical process involving the separation of small molecules in solution from larger ones, through a separating (or dialysing) membrane.

Ultrafiltration

The filtration function of this membrane means that cells and large molecules are retained in the capillaries while smaller molecules are able to pass into the capsular space. This is a process of filtration on a small scale so it is called ultrafiltration. Blood cells, platelets and large plasma

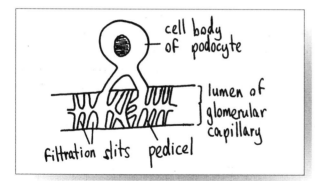

Diagram 9.6 An individual podocyte forms a physical filter around a length of glomerular capillary. The branches of the podocyte form a very fine physical sieve over the surface of the glomerular capillaries.

Diagram 9.7 The three layers of the endothelial-capsular membrane: capillary endothelial cells, the basement membrane and filtration slits between branches of the podocyte. Arrows indicate the direction of filtrate formation, from the glomerular capillaries into the glomerular capsular space.

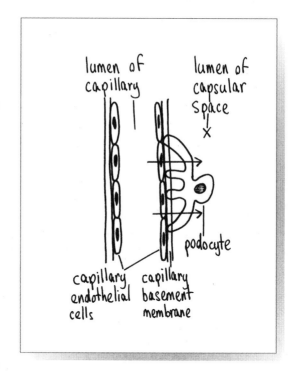

proteins are retained while smaller molecules such as water, glucose, urea, amino acids, sodium, potassium and creatine pass into the filtrate.

Glomerular filtration rate refers to the volume of filtrate formed. This is about 125 ml per minute, which adds up to 180 litres per day. Filtrate is formed as a result of blood pressure in the glomerular capillaries pushing water and solutes through the endothelial-capsular membrane into the capsular space ('solute' just means a substance dissolved in solution, in this case in the blood plasma). Once in the capsular space filtrate is free to pass along the rest of the renal tubule.

The need for an adequate blood pressure to generate filtrate explains why acute renal failure may be a complication of shock. In shock there is a low systemic blood pressure; if the systolic BP falls below 80 mm Hg, glomerular filtration rate will start to decline.

Tubular reabsorption

As glomerular filtrate passes through the nephron, as much as 99% is reabsorbed back into the blood. This is why the efferent arteriole breaks down into a network of capillaries that carry on to surround the tubule. Material is reabsorbed from the tubules into the capillary network. Blood containing reabsorbed material is then collected in a venule that drains into a branch of the renal vein. Cell surfaces lining much of the lumen of the renal tubules are infolded into microvilli that form a brush border. This infolding greatly increases the internal surface area available over which reabsorption may take place.

From the glomerular space, filtrate enters the renal tubule and passes around the proximal convoluted tubule and on into the loop of the nephron. As filtrate passes through the tubule, material is progressively reabsorbed. After the distal convoluted tubule the fluid remaining in the nephron passes into the collecting duct. Collecting ducts originate in the cortex where they are small; however, as they pass

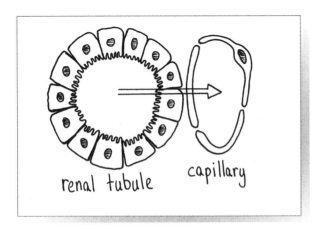

Diagram 9.8 Cross-section of a renal tubule and adjacent capillary. Reabsorption occurs from the renal tubules back into the capillaries. Arrow indicates direction of flow.

renal tubule   capillary

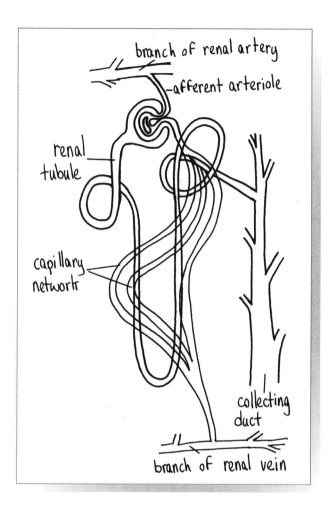

branch of renal artery

afferent arteriole

renal tubule

capillary network

collecting duct

branch of renal vein

Diagram 9.9 The relationship between the tubule and capillary network. Capillaries wrap around the renal tubule to allow reabsorption to occur efficiently over short distances. (This diagram is much clearer if you colour in the filtrate in the nephron and then the blood in the capillaries.) Only three capillaries are illustrated.

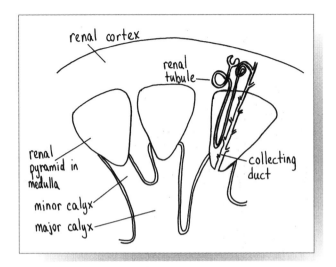

Diagram 9.10 These two diagrams illustrate the relationship between the microscopic and macroscopic structure of the kidney. Any filtrate that is not reabsorbed passes from the collecting ducts into the renal pelvis.

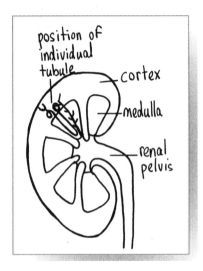

down through the medulla they merge into progressively larger ducts that eventually drain from the apex of the medullary pyramids into the renal pelvis. Any filtrate which is not reabsorbed is left as urine. Some reabsorption takes place from the collecting ducts; however, once urine is passed into the renal pelvis no further reabsorption is possible.

Selective reabsorption and homeostasis

Reabsorption from the tubule is selective. Materials that the body needs – such as glucose and amino acids – are totally reabsorbed. In health, urine should contain no sugar or amino acids at all. Other substances are not extensively reabsorbed, and therefore enter the urine. Chemicals that are not reabsorbed include urea and creatine, both of which contain toxic wastes generated in metabolic processes.

Other substances are reabsorbed depending on the body's requirements at the time. For example, if we drink a lot, it will be necessary to reabsorb less water from the nephrons. If less water is reabsorbed, more will remain in the tubules and pass into the collecting ducts. This will have the effect of increasing urine volumes, excreting the excess water. Conversely, if someone has not been able to drink for a period of time, the blood will become more concentrated and it will be necessary to conserve water. To achieve this more water will be reabsorbed from the nephron; this will leave less in the tubules so less will pass into the collecting ducts. This will lower urine volumes, conserving water in the body.

In addition to water, there are other substances that are selectively reabsorbed depending on the body's current requirements. For example, levels of sodium and potassium must be homeostatically controlled in the blood. If we eat a lot of salty food (salt is sodium chloride) less sodium is reabsorbed, so more is excreted. The amount of sodium that is reabsorbed is controlled by the levels of the hormone aldosterone. As plasma levels of aldosterone rise so does reabsorption of sodium.

It is particularly important that serum potassium levels are finely controlled. If these rise or fall too much the electrical functioning of the myocardium may be affected, causing cardiac arrest. Diets high in potassium will increase the amount of potassium found in the urine. Conversely, if the diet is low in potassium less will be excreted in urine. Water-soluble vitamins may also be selectively reabsorbed. If we eat too much vitamin C less is reabsorbed so vitamin C will be found in the urine.

The kidneys are also the principle route for excretion of drugs from the body. After taking a particular drug the metabolites will be found in urine. A drug metabolite is a breakdown product of a drug. Drug metabolism usually takes place in the liver. Renal excretion explains why we need to be careful when giving drugs to patients with poor renal function. If the body cannot excrete a drug in urine, it may build up to toxic levels.

Mechanisms of reabsorption

There are basically two mechanisms by which material is reabsorbed from the renal tubules. The first is a passive reabsorption via the mechanisms of diffusion and osmosis. Water will move from areas of high water concentration in the first part of the tubule back into the blood, where the concentration of water is relatively lower. Other substances will also diffuse from filtrate back to the blood, down their diffusional concentration gradients. However, whenever reabsorption is required against a diffusion gradient, active transport mechanisms must be used. These are mostly membrane-based systems that use energy to pump substances from the tubule where they are at relatively low concentrations into the blood, where their concentrations are already relatively high.

Active transport explains why there are normally no glucose or amino acids at all in urine. It is true that in the proximal sections of the renal tubules there may be passive reabsorption of these nutrients, when the concentrations in filtrate are greater than those in the blood. However, in the distal sections, much of the glucose and amino acids have already been reabsorbed. This will have increased the concentrations in the blood while reducing concentrations left in filtrate; this will generate a diffusion gradient from blood to filtrate. This means in order to reabsorb all glucose and amino acids, the remaining molecules must be pumped from the filtrate into the blood against their diffusion gradients.

Plasma is 'cleaned' 60 times a day

As plasma volume is only about 3 litres, the high volumes of glomerular filtration and selective reabsorption means that the entire plasma is cleansed of impurities and homeostatically regulated about 60 times per day. This allows for very fine ongoing homeostatic regulation of numerous constituents of the blood and prevents us feeling ill as a result of toxin accumulation.

Tubular secretion

In the process of tubular secretion material is transferred directly from the blood capillaries into the lumen of the tubules. This is the opposite direction to the flow of materiel in reabsorption. Waste products such as ammonia are excreted in this way, as are some drugs. Potassium and hydrogen ions are selectively secreted by tubular secretion, depending on the body's current homeostatic requirements. If we eat a lot of bananas, for example, serum potassium will start to rise. In this case, tubular secretion of potassium will be increased, and this will result in more being excreted in urine. Material secreted from the blood into filtrate will carry on through the renal tubule, into the collecting duct and enter the renal pelvis as a component of urine. Active transport mechanisms are usually used to facilitate tubular secretion.

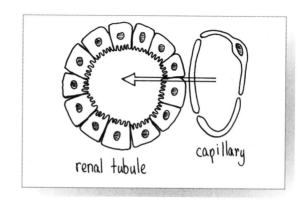

Diagram 9.11 Cross section of a renal tubule and adjacent capillary. Tubular secretion occurs in the opposite direction to reabsorption. Arrow indicates direction of flow.

Essential science

Acids and alkalis

The strength of an acidic solution is determined by the number of free hydrogen ions (H^+) in solution, stronger acids having more. An alkaline solution is able to absorb hydrogen ions, for example, the hydroxyl ion (OH^-) can absorb an H^+ to form water.

In physiology it is vital to maintain plasma pH levels within finely turned parameters. This is because all metabolic biochemical processes are facilitated by enzymes and enzymes are very sensitive to small changes in pH. If the pH falls or rises, enzymic function would be rapidly and potentially fatally affected.

The pH of the blood is partly controlled by regulation of the number of hydrogen ions in plasma. An increase in H^+ concentration increases acidity. When the pH of the blood falls and acidity rises, there will be more tubular secretion of hydrogen ions, which will reduce the H^+ concentration in the blood while increasing the concentration in urine. As a result of this, blood pH will rise back to normal as acidity reduces.

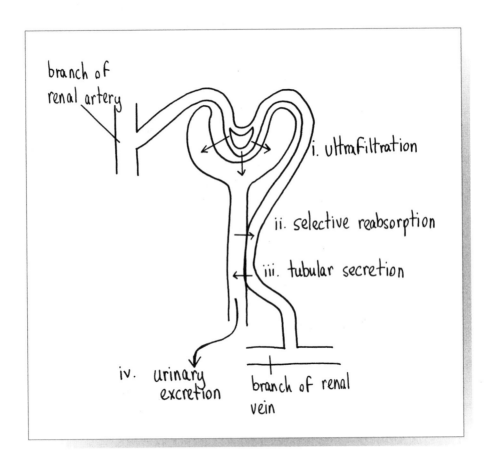

Diagram 9.12 Summary of the four functions of a nephron:
(i) ultrafiltration;
(ii) selective tubular reabsorption;
(iii) tubular secretion;
(iv) urine excretion.

Urine

Normal urine

Typically urine is about 95% water and 5% dissolved substances or solutes. Because urine contains these solutes it is more dense than pure water; a normal specific gravity of urine is about 1.010–1.035. (Specific gravity describes the mass of a substance as a ratio to the mass of pure water.) Solutes are derived from metabolic processes, the diet and sometimes from drugs, normally as metabolites.

Metabolism of amino acids results in the formation of waste nitrogen. This chemically combines with water to form ammonia, which is toxic. In order to rapidly remove this toxic waste from the blood, the liver facilitates a chemical reaction that combines ammonia with carbon dioxide to form less toxic urea. As urea is very soluble in water it may easily be excreted in urine. Creatine and uric acid are other nitrogen-containing wastes. Levels of nitrogen excretion will increase if more protein is eaten as proteins contain nitrogen in addition to carbon, hydrogen and oxygen.

Other normal constituents present in various amounts are sodium, potassium, magnesium, calcium, sulphate, chlorides and phosphates. Normal urine may also contain some ketones, especially if the person has not been eating much in the recent past. Ketones are breakdown products of fat metabolism.

Normal urine should be transparent; if it is cloudy this may indicate the presence of bacteria. Urine is normally a yellow to amber colour; the more concentrated the urine the darker the colour. The colour comes from a breakdown produce of bile called urochrome. Urine is normally slightly acidic. Diets rich in protein tend to increase acidity, and vegetarian diets cause an increase in alkalinity.

Urine volumes

The volumes and constituents of urine will vary significantly depending on the excretory needs of the time. Most adults produce between 1 and 2 litres of urine per day. It is a good idea to drink water from time to time during the day to maintain good urine volumes. This will mean urine produced is more dilute and will be passed more often. Dilute urine may reduce the risk of precipitation in the urinary tract.

Precipitation (i.e. formation of solids from solutions) can lead to the formation of very painful and troublesome kidney and bladder stones. Larger urine volumes will also physically flush out the ureters, bladder and urethra, reducing the probability of urinary infections. Urinary tract infections (UTIs) are common in women owing to the short urethra and proximity of the anus. These infections commonly present as inflammation of the bladder or cystitis.

This flushing effect of larger urine volumes may also help to wash out potential carcinogens. The presence of cancer-causing chemicals in urine may be caused by smoking. Some of the toxins from smoke pass from the lungs into the blood and are then excreted by the kidneys. This may explain why smokers are more at risk of renal and bladder cancers than non-smokers.

Tea, coffee and alcohol are all diuretics. (A diuretic is any agent that will increase urine volumes.) Diuretics result in larger volumes of urine than would be expected from the volume of fluids consumed. Diuresis therefore results in subsequent dehydration and production of smaller volumes of more concentrated urine. Drinking water as well as these other drinks will help to compensate for their diuretic effects.

Obligatory urine volume

The kidney is able to alter the volumes of water excreted without altering the volumes of waste products excreted. When urine volumes are low, urea, creatine, excess sodium and potassium can still be excreted. However, there is a limit to the kidney's ability to concentrate these wastes. This means that when urine volumes drop below a critical level, the body is no longer excreting all the waste material it needs to. Clearly this will result in waste accumulation and the development of toxic effects. For an average 70 kg adult this minimum urine obligatory volume is 500 ml; any less and toxins will be retained. This gives a rationale for a common definition of acute renal failure, which is 'when less than 20 ml of urine are produced per hour for two consecutive hours'. (We can only know this if the patient is catheterized.)

The limits to urine concentration have important implications if you are ever lost at sea with limited supplies of fresh water. In this situation, it would be best not to drink any of your water supply until the kidneys are concentrating urine to their maximum ability. After this you should just drink enough to produce the obligatory volume. This will preserve water supplies, but prevent you from becoming toxic.

It is always harmful to drink any sea water, as this is already more concentrated than the most concentrated urine the kidneys can produce. One litre of sea water needs 2 litres of urine volume to excrete the salt it contains.

Abnormal urine

Urinalysis should be performed on every patient assessed by nurses. It is a quick, safe, cheap non-invasive screen for several possible disorders. Presence of the following substances is always abnormal: protein, glucose and blood. Proteinuria (protein in the urine) may indicate damage to the glomerular membrane caused by disease or high blood pressure. Glucoseuria indicates that the levels of glucose in the blood are too high suggesting the possibility of diabetes mellitus. Haematuria may derive from any part of the tract and may be caused by trauma or neoplasm (possibly cancer) but more commonly infection. Contamination from menstruation is also common and, of course, normal; just check the urine again in the following week, after menstruation has finished. High levels of ketones may indicate the person has not been eating or has diabetes mellitus.

Homeostasis of blood pressure

As the kidneys regulate the amounts of water and salts in the blood they are a major factor in determining venous return to the heart. Venous return influences cardiac output, which is a principal determinant of blood pressure. If the kidneys retain more water, venous return will be increased. If they excrete more water, venous return will be reduced. When more sodium is retained the osmotic pressure of plasma is increased; this in turn attracts more water into the circulation, increasing plasma volume and venous return. If more salt is excreted, however, plasma sodium will be reduced, lowering the osmotic pressure of the plasma and so lowering plasma volumes.

Juxtaglomerular apparatus

This is located next to the glomerulus ('juxta-' means 'beside'). Juxtaglomerular (JG) cells are located in the wall of the afferent arteriole close to the point at which it divides into the capillaries of the glomerulus. These cells are able to monitor the blood pressure in the arteriole; they also produce and store renin. If blood pressure drops, JG cells respond by secreting renin into the blood.

One of the proteins present in the blood is called angiotensinogen. This is a short protein produced by the liver and is inactive – it just circulates in the blood. However, when renin acts on angiotensinogen it converts it into another shorter protein called angiotensin I. As angiotensin I passes through the lungs it is converted into angiotensin II by an enzyme called angiotensin converting enzyme (ACE). Angiotensin II is a powerful vascular vasoconstrictor; this will increase peripheral resistance which will in turn increase blood pressure.

If the systemic blood pressure is increased the pressure in the afferent arteriole will also be increased. This will be detected by the JGA cells, which will respond by stopping renin secretion. When renin is not present in the blood, angiotensinogen will remain in inactive form. This renin–angiotensin mechanism allows the kidneys to regulate their own blood flow to an extent; when an organ regulates itself in this way it is called autoregulation.

You may have come across ACE-inhibiting drugs; these inhibit ACE and so inhibit the conversion of angiotensin I into angiotensin II. If there is less angiotensin II there will be less vasoconstriction so blood pressure will be lowered.

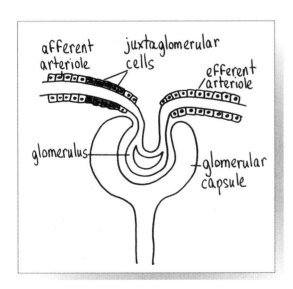

Diagram 9.13
Juxtaglomerular apparatus.

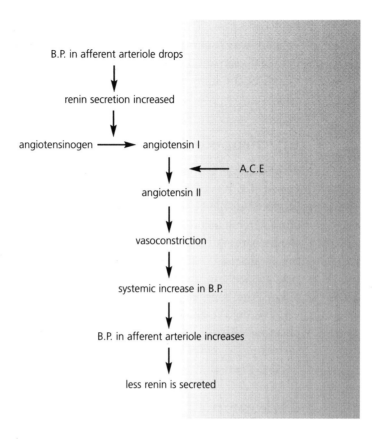

B.P. in afferent arteriole drops

↓

renin secretion increased

↓

angiotensinogen ——————▶ angiotensin I

↓ ◀—————— A.C.E

angiotensin II

↓

vasoconstriction

↓

systemic increase in B.P.

↓

B.P. in afferent arteriole increases

↓

less renin is secreted

Table 9.1 Regulation of blood pressure via the renin–angiotensin mechanism.

Renal endocrine functions

Activation of vitamin D

Vitamin D eaten in the diet or generated by the skin when exposed to sunlight is in the form of vitamin D_3 (cholecalciferol). This form of the vitamin is almost completely physiologically inactive; however, in the kidneys it is converted into an active form called calcitriol. This form is 1000 times more active than the D_3 form. Conversion is actually facilitated by an enzyme produced in the proximal tubules. Activated vitamin D (i.e. calcitriol) increases calcium absorption from the gut and influences calcium metabolism in the bones by increasing bone deposition. This function of the kidneys in activating vitamin D explains why patients with chronic renal failure lose bone mass. Many people classify calcitriol as an endocrine hormone because it is generated in the kidney, passes into the blood and affects other target tissues.

Erythropoietin

This is an endocrine hormone produced by the kidneys and is discussed in Chapter 3. Normally 90% of circulating erythropoietin is produced in the kidney; the remaining 10% comes from the liver. In chronic renal failure, this remaining 10% is not sufficient to stimulate the formation of enough erythrocytes, resulting in the development of severe anaemia. Although erythropoietin is a large glycoprotein it is now available in injectable form. When given to patients with renal failure, the bone marrow is able to produce normal amounts of red cells, curing the anaemia. In recent years, this 'epo' has been used by cheating athletes to increase the number of red cells in their blood, so increasing its oxygen-carrying and aerobic capacity. It is currently unclear where in the kidney erythropoietin is produced.

The urinary tract

The urinary tract begins in the kidneys when minor calyces join together to form major calyces that merge to form the renal pelvis. From here the urinary tract has a continuous surface down the ureters, through the bladder to the urethra. The inner lining of the tract is referred to as the mucosa. This is a mucous membrane, lined with a layer of mucus, and composed of transitional epithelium. Mucus lining protects the cells of the epithelium from the urine within the lumen of the tract.

Ureters

The right and left ureter are continuous with the right and left renal pelvis. They pass down for about 30 cm, behind the peritoneum of the abdominal cavity and join the posterior, inferior aspect of the bladder.

Ureteric lumen is lined with mucosa; this is a mucous membrane that secretes a layer of mucus to protect the transitional epithelial cells from urine.

Under the mucosa is a muscular layer containing outer circular and inner longitudinal smooth muscle fibres. These facilitate peristaltic waves of contraction from the renal pelvis down to the bladder. The peristaltic nature of the ureter is an important mechanism preventing urine from the bladder regurgitating back into the renal pelvis. It is important this does not happen as infection could ascend to the kidneys causing nephritis. Peristalsis of the ureters further allows the bladder to fill when we are lying flat or are positioned head down.

The outer layer of the ureters is composed of fibrous connective tissue; this secures the position relative to other structures to prevent kinks.

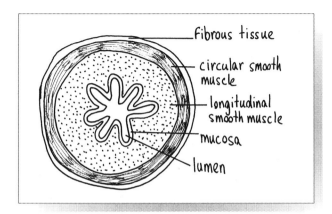

Diagram 9.14
Cross-section of a ureter.

Urinary bladder

This structure is located on the floor of the pelvic cavity. In women it is just in front of the vagina, and in men it is in front of the rectum. It is essentially a muscular sac that stores urine until it can be voided. Mucosa lining the bladder is arranged in folds when the bladder is empty; these allow stretching as the bladder fills. The smooth muscle of the bladder wall is called the detrusor muscle.

Passing urine

Micturition is the emptying of the bladder. When the detrusor muscle contracts it increases the pressure of urine stored in the bladder. When accompanied by relaxation of the sphincter between the bladder and urethra, urine will be expelled. Stimulation by sympathetic nerves causes retention of urine by relaxing the detrusor muscle while contracting the sphincter. This is why it is sometimes difficult to pass urine when we feel anxious. Passage of urine is facilitated by parasympathetic stimulation; this will contract the detrusor while relaxing the sphincter.

This sphincter discussed above is under autonomic control and is located at the base of the bladder around the area where the urethra leaves. However, there is a second sphincter a little way along the urethra. This sphincter is referred to as the external sphincter and is under voluntary control. It is the presence of the external voluntary sphincter that allows us to initiate and stop the flow of urine under control of our will. In women, most of the action of the external sphincter is provided by the pelvic floor muscles. This is why female continence of urine can be improved by pelvic floor muscle exercises. In men, the voluntary muscle sphincter forms part of the urethral wall.

Bladder wall contains stretch receptors that alert the individual to bladder filling. Micturition often occurs when the bladder contains 280 ml of urine. If it is inconvenient to pass urine, up to 500 ml may be retained but beyond this discomfort or pain is experienced.

The activity of a voluntary external sphincter explains why people may be incontinent of urine if they become unconscious, such as during an epileptic fit. This is also why patients are asked to empty their bladder before being anaesthetized. All babies are incontinent of urine because the nervous connections to the external sphincter are not fully developed. When the bladder is distended to a certain point, a micturition reflex is stimulated. After the age of about 2 years, the nervous connections to the external sphincter are usually developed, allowing control of micturition to be learned.

Prevention of reflux

In addition to unidirectional peristalsis, reflux of urine from the bladder, back into the ureters is aided by the ureters entering the bladder inferiorly. As the bladder fills up the wall is stretched, leading to an increase in volume and size. This means that the fuller the bladder is, the more pressure it will impose on the distal sections of the ureters. This increase in pressure will prevent reflux of urine from a full or filling bladder.

Diagram 9.15 Urinary bladder in a man. (In women there is no prostate gland and the external sphincter is mostly provided by pelvic floor muscles external to the urethra).

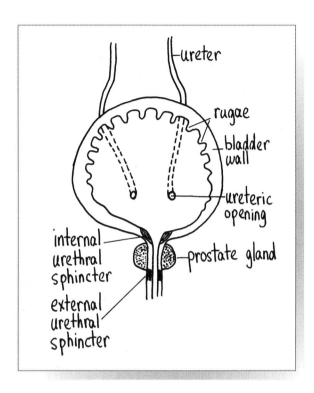

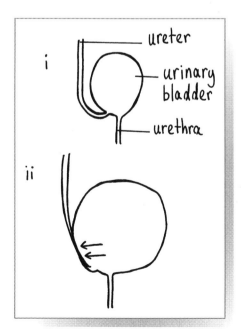

Diagram 9.16
(i) The anatomical relationship of the ureter and an empty bladder.
(ii) When the bladder is full it exerts a pressure on the ureters preventing reflux of potentially infected urine into the ureter. Arrows indicate direction of pressure on the distal ureter.

Urethra

Urine is drained from the bladder to the outside world via the urethra. In men the urethra is about 18–20 cm long. The first 3–4 cm of the male urethra passes through the tissue of the prostate gland. This is why the lumen of the urethra is compressed if the prostate gland enlarges; if this occurs the stream of urine becomes thin and difficult to initiate. The urethra passes through the penis to an opening at the end called the urethral meatus.

Diagram 9.17 The urinary bladder and path of the urethra in a man.

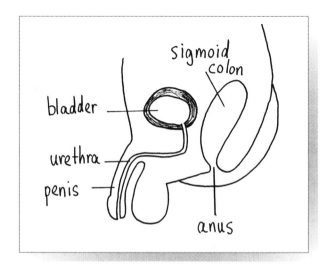

In females the urethra is about 4 cm long. After leaving the bladder it travels in the anterior wall of the vagina. The urethral orifice is anterior to the vagina, about 2.5 cm inferior to the clitoris. When no urine is passing the urethra is a closed slit; this helps to prevent infection ascending into the bladder from the outside. Despite this, the relatively short length of the urethra and its proximity to the anus means that women are more prone to infections of the bladder than men.

CHAPTER 10

The skin

Skin covers the entire outer surface of the body and is continuous with the membranes that line the various orifices such as the mouth, anus and vagina. Skin thickness varies over different parts of the body from about 1.5 to 4 mm. In an average adult it accounts for 8% of body mass. This means that in terms of mass the skin is the largest organ in the body. The second largest is the liver which is normally less than 3% of body mass. Clearly, skin surface area varies between individuals, but in most adults it covers about 1.5 to 2 square metres. Skin is arranged in two distinct layers, the outer epidermis and, underlying this, the dermis.

Epidermis

Epidermis does not contain blood or lymphatic vessels. It is nourished and oxygenated by diffusion via the tissue fluid of the dermis.

Epidermal–dermal junction

The junction between the two layers of the skin is undulating, with numerous projections from the epidermis dipping down into the dermis. This allows for a great deal of resistance to shearing forces, preventing epidermis being rubbed away from dermis. When this does happen, e.g. as a result of persistent friction, a blister results. A blister is a collection of fluid between the dermis and epidermis. Under a light microscope, the epidermal–dermal junction is marked by a basement membrane; with the higher power of an electron microscope this is seen to be incomplete. This is why the junction between the epidermis and dermis is correctly referred to as the basement membrane zone.

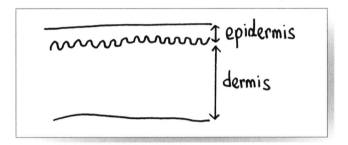

Diagram 10.1 There are two distinct layers in the skin as seen in this cross-section.

Epidermal turnover

Living epidermal cells are positioned on the basement membrane zone. This area is often called the germinative layer, because there is on-going mitosis in epidermal cells. Epidermal cells are correctly referred to as keratinocytes. Approximately 10% of keratinocytes are epidermal stem cells. These stem cells divide, producing one further stem cell and another keratinocyte. Once formed, these keratinocytes are capable of a limited number of further mitotic divisions. When young, keratinocytes are usually cuboidal to columnar in shape. As mitosis is ongoing, young cells push older ones upwards, away from the germinative layer on the basement membrane zone. Because epidermal cells are nourished and oxygenated from the tissue fluid of the dermis, they become progressively hypoxic the further they are pushed upwards. This means only the cells near the bottom of the epidermis are alive; the outer layers are composed of dead cells.

This turnover of cells from the deeper layers of epidermis to the surface means the upper layer of the skin is constantly being regenerated. Complete turnover time for the epidermis is typically about 8 weeks; the best quoted figure is 52–75 days, depending on the individual and on the site on the body surface. Once dead keratin-rich cells reach the surface, they are shed. You may have noticed an accumulation of white material on the skin surface when towelling yourself down after a shower. This is in fact a collection of dead keratinocytes. Most of the dust that accumulates in our houses is dead human epidermal cells.

Stratified, keratinized, squamous, epithelium

These four terms concisely describe the epidermis. Stratified indicates the epidermis is composed of several layers of cells. Stratification allows the skin to resist external forces. If some epidermis is removed it can rapidly be replaced from underlying cells.

Keratin is a hard, dry, horny protein. Hair and fingernails are mostly keratin. By the time the keratinocytes reach the surface of the epidermis they are composed largely of keratin. Keratin keeps the outer layer of epidermis fairly hard and able to resist friction and trauma. Cells in the basal, germinative layer of the epidermis do contain some keratin; as the keratinocytes near the surface, however, the amounts of keratin increase. Proteins from the cell cytoplasm are progressively converted into keratin as they rise to the epidermal surface.

Squamous refers to the flattened appearance of the upper skin cells. As the columnar and cuboidal keratinocytes are pushed away from the germinative layer they are subject to pressure from the skin surface. This means the cells are progressively flattened and adopt a squamous appearance.

Epidermis is an epithelium because it is a tissue that lines the surface of the body.

Epidermal lipids

Keratinocytes secrete a variety of lipids, particularly in the upper layers of the epidermis. These help to hold the individual cells together, rather like cement holding bricks together in a wall. In addition, because the lipids are oily they repel water (remember lipids are

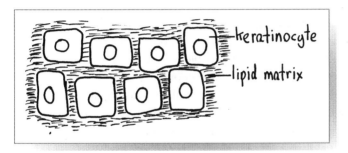

Diagram 10.2 Individual keratinocytes are held together by a lipid matrix.

hydrophobic); this is part of the reason skin is waterproof. We all know it is important for us to wash our hands between patients at work; however, repeated washing with soap degrades the natural oils in skin and causes it to 'dry out', which can in turn lead to cracking and soreness. Bacteria may colonize these cracks in our skin, ironically making cross-infection more likely. Moisturizing creams may partly compensate for loss of natural skin lipids.

Synthesis of vitamin D

One of the lipid-based molecules found in the epidermis is called dehydrocholesterol. When this substance is exposed to sunlight it is converted into a form of vitamin D. In people who have diets deficient in vitamin D, this mechanism is essential to prevent deficiency. In children, lack of vitamin D causes rickets.

Epidermal melanocytes

Melanin is the pigment found in the epidermis that gives skin colour. White people have small amounts of melanin. The darker a shade of brown or black a person is, the more melanin is present. The red and yellow colours in human skin characteristic of some races are generated by a second form of melanin. Melanocytes are a specialized form of cell found in the epidermis; they synthesize and secrete melanin. In order to aid distribution of melanin to the epidermis, melanocytes contain projections called dendrites.

　　Sunlight contains potentially harmful ultraviolet (UV) radiation; it is the function of melanin to absorb this to protect underlying tissues. Exposure to sunlight therefore increases melanin synthesis rates and causes the skin to darken. However, the process of increasing melanin synthesis takes a few weeks to a few months to fully develop. Before there is sufficient melanin to protect the skin, the melanocytes are themselves prone to UV damage. After a winter in the UK melanin levels for white-skinned people will be low; if they then fly off to a sunny country they will not have enough melanin to protect their skin against UV radiation. This can result in burning and damage to the DNA of the melanocytes. Some forms of DNA damage can lead to cancer. Malignant melanoma is cancer of a melanocyte line and can spread very rapidly.

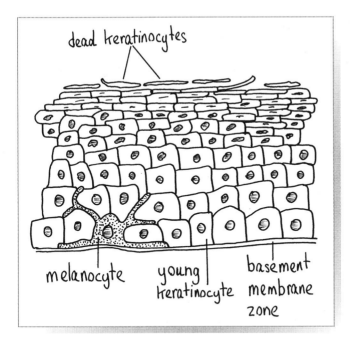

Diagram 10.3 Cross-section of the
epidermis. Dead keratin-rich keratinocytes
are shed from the skin surface.

Dermis

The dermis is a connective tissue that contains several types of
structures such as hair follicles, sebaceous glands, sweat glands, nerve
endings, blood and lymphatic vessels.

Collagen

There are several forms of collagen protein, which forms long strands and
often occurs in bundles. Collagen has high tensile strength, making it
very hard to snap. It is the presence of collagen that gives skin internal
strength and prevents it becoming detached from underlying tissues. You
may have noticed that the elderly are more prone to injuries where some
skin is rubbed off. This occurs because old skin contains relatively less
collagen than young skin. Collagen also provides a three-dimensional
structure that gives the skin 'body'.

Elastic fibres

Skin is very elastic, and it may be stretched to a degree when closing wounds. Elasticity is also demonstrated over joints and during pregnancy. Elastic fibres running throughout the dermis give the skin this useful property.

Fibroblasts

Fibroblasts are found throughout the dermis, and produce the collagen and elastic fibres. In addition, the dermis contains a protein-based ground substance called proteoglycan, which is also probably mostly derived from fibroblasts.

Hair follicles

Hair grows out of structures called follicles. These are downward projections of the epidermis, penetrating into the dermis and sometimes subcutaneous tissues. The outer layer of the follicle is composed of a fibrous sheath. Within this is a layer of epidermal tissue. At the base of the follicle is a layer of actively dividing epidermal cells forming an area called the hair bulb. As epidermal cells divide, older ones are pushed away from their dermal nutrient and oxygen source and so die. Further mitosis pushes the already-dead keratinized cells further up the follicle forming a hair shaft. Melanocytes at the base of the bulb produce pigmented melanin that gives hair colour. There is a capillary loop at the base of each hair bulb to oxygenate and nourish the actively dividing epidermal cells.

The presence of epidermal protrusions down into the dermis and subcutaneous tissues, as found in hair follicles, has important implications for wound healing. If the epidermis and part of the dermis is lost due to trauma or a burn, epidermal tissue is able to regenerate from below, by mitosis of surviving keratinocyte germ cells. This allows partial thickness wounds to heal without scarring. In this context partial thickness means part way through the dermis. The same principle of healing allows the donor site of a skin graft to heal rapidly with minimal or no scarring.

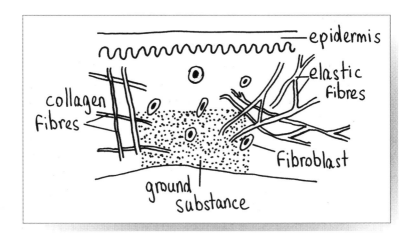

Diagram 10.4 Diagrammatic representation of the principal structural components of the dermis.

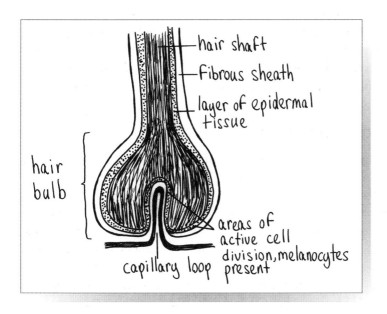

Diagram 10.5 The growing area of a hair in a follicle.

Hair

Hair of varying lengths and thickness grow from all of the skin surface except the palms, soles and lower surfaces of the fingers and toes. Hair follicles are well innervated with sensory nerve fibres. This means hair increases the sensitivity of the skin to light stimuli. In the nose, hairs are able to trap inhaled foreign material such as insects. Eyelashes are very sensitive and may initiate reflex closure of the eyelids as a protective measure. Hair on the head helps to protect from sunlight.

The presence of hair near the skin surface generates a boundary layer of air. This is a layer of air that remains relatively static over the surface of the body. As air is an excellent insulator of heat, a boundary layer helps to prevent body cooling in cold environments. This mechanism works better in more hairy people.

Hair erector muscles (usually called arrector pili) are small bundles of smooth muscle connected to the fibrous capsule of the hair follicles. When these muscles contract they cause the hair to stand in an erect position. This has the effect of increasing the depth of the boundary layer and so occurs in response to cold. Another consequence of this contraction is the production of numerous small indentations over the skin surface, often referred to as 'goose pimples'.

Distribution of hair growth is partly determined by the concentrations of oestrogen and testosterone in the blood. This gives rise to different distributions in body hair between men and women.

Sebaceous glands

These glands are lined with specialized secretory cells that produce sebum. Once secreted, this passes along a small duct into the hair follicle. From here, sebum moves towards the skin surface. There may be several sebaceous units associated with a single follicle. Sebum is a lipid-based oily substance that coats the hair and skin surface, helping to keep it moist and supple. Because it is oily, sebum aids in the waterproofing of skin. Around the time of puberty, in both males and females, hormonal influences increase the size of sebaceous glands and sebum production. Excessive production of sebum may lead to impaction in the sebaceous ducts. This causes stasis and subsequent infection and is the main cause of acne.

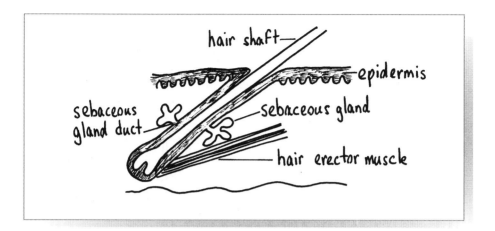

Diagram 10.6 Hair follicle showing the relationship between the hair, follicle, hair erector muscle, sebaceous gland and duct.

Sweat glands

Glands that produce sweat are essentially long, unbranched tubes. The common form of sweat glands are correctly termed eccrine glands. Sweat is produced in the lower coiled part of the gland and passes up to the surface of the skin via a duct. There are approximately 2–4 million sweat glands in the skin; numbers vary between individuals for genetic reasons. Races from hotter countries usually have more sweat glands than people from temperate zones. Like hair follicles, sweat gland ducts are lined with epidermal cells. Sweat is produced in response to a rise in body temperature; this mechanism is controlled via the hypothalamus. Anxiety and other emotions also cause sweating because the glands are stimulated by the sympathetic nervous system. This is why we can get a 'cold sweat' when anxious.

Sweat is a clear odourless fluid. In addition to water it contains salt (sodium and chloride ions) with some potassium, urea, and other

Diagram 10.7
Sweat gland.

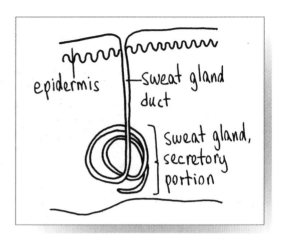

trace substances. In extreme circumstances the body's sweat glands are capable of producing 10 litres of sweat per day.

There is a second form of sweat gland called an apocrine gland. These are found primarily in the axilla, groin and around the genitalia. Apocrine ducts open into hair follicles. These glands start to function at puberty in males and females, under hormonal influences. Once on the skin surface some of the components in apocrine sweat are degraded by bacteria. It is these breakdown products that cause unwashed armpits and groins to smell. Some people have suggested that these smells, or other breakdown products that we cannot consciously smell, act as pheromones, generating sexual interest in potential partners. You can make your own mind up on that one.

Nerve endings

The skin is the principle organ of tactility (the sense of feeling). There are basically four types of sensation that the skin detects; these are light touch, pressure, temperature and pain. Sensations are generated by peripheral sensory receptors. These convert a tactile stimulus into a series of nerve impulses that are relayed to the sensory areas of the brain via sensory neurones. The brain interprets these electrical impulses to generate the appropriate sensations that we then experience.

Specialized structures called Messner's receptors, located just under the epidermis, are sensitive to touch. When touch is detected they generate a sensory nerve impulse. There are also a few touch receptors just above the basement membrane in the lower area of the epidermis; these are called Merkel-cell receptors. These same Merkel-type detectors also innervate hair follicles so we can detect touch from hairs. The combination of these detectors allows for skin to be superbly sensitive to the lightest of touch. Touch receptors are particularly common in the fingertips, eyelids, lips, penis and clitoris.

Sensations of pressure are generated by large receptors deep in the dermis. These are referred to as pacinian corpuscles. Pressure awareness allows us to hold objects with an appropriate degree of force. This is important to stop us from dropping tools or crushing eggs.

Thermoreceptors detect changes in temperature; for example, when we get into cold water it feels cold at first, then we get used to it. This is because once the temperature is no longer changing we are not so aware of it. There are two types of temperature detectors in the dermis. Cold receptors detect a drop in skin temperature and warm receptors detect an increase. Because these receptors are located throughout the dermis, we can detect the temperature of localized areas of skin surface, as well as overall ambient temperature. Thermoreceptors are probably specialized free nerve endings in the

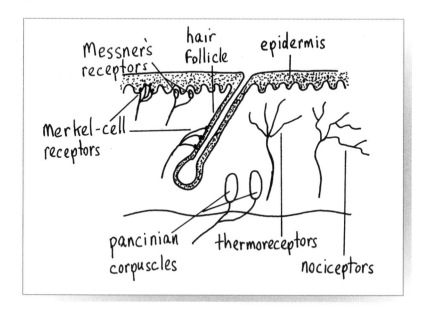

Diagram 10.8 The sense of tactility, detection of touch, pressure, temperature and pain.

dermis – they do not have an anatomically recognizable receptor like touch and pressure receptors have.

Pain is detected by specialist neurones that respond only to pain. These are definitely only free nerve endings in the dermis. They are correctly referred to as nociceptors. Pain detection is nociception, the detection of the noxious. Fortunately, pain receptors only generate an impulse in response to trauma or to being cut.

Pain is essential to prevent the tissues of the body being damaged. It also promotes rest if an area of the body has been damaged, for example we do not go running on a sprained ankle. Perhaps the value of pain can be most clearly seen when it is absent. People with Hanson's disease (leprosy) often burn their hands picking up hot cooking pots, because they cannot feel the pain. A similar situation may occur in peripheral sensory neuropathy, a long-term complication of diabetes. Because these patients cannot feel pain from their feet they suffer from pressure effects that lead on to tissue damage and infection.

Blood vessels

Small arteries deep in the dermis sub divide into numerous small arterioles. These arterioles in turn perfuse large numbers of capillaries. Capillaries drain into venules that drain into small veins. The amount of blood flowing through the dermis may be controlled by increasing or reducing the volumes flowing through the capillary beds. Before each bed of capillaries there is a ring of muscle, located in the arteriole wall, called the pre-capillary sphincter. If the pre-capillary sphincter contracts, this will reduce the lumen of the arteriole and so limit the volume of blood passing into the capillary bed. However, if the sphincter relaxes, the arteriole will get wider which will increase the flow of blood through the dermal capillaries. Contraction of the pre-capillary sphincter causes peripheral vasoconstriction and relaxation causes vasodilation.

Dermal capillaries also form, and largely reabsorb tissue fluid; this is essential to provide a diffusional medium for both dermal and lower epidermal cells.

Lymphatic vessels

The dermis is drained by lymphatic capillaries that drain into larger lymphatic vessels as discussed in Chapter 5.

Hypodermis

Below the dermis is a subcutaneous layer sometimes referred to as the hypodermis. This varies in thickness over different parts of the body and between individuals. It contains mostly adipose tissue with varying amounts of connective fibres.

Age-related changes

Overall skin condition deteriorates with age; this affects both the epidermis and dermis. As is probably the case with all body tissues, two factors contribute to age-related changes – chronological and environmental. Chronological factors occur as a result of ageing but show considerable variation between individuals. The reasons why some people appear to 'age better' than others are not fully understood but are probably mostly related to genetic make-up.

Environmental ageing of skin is primarily a consequence of chronic exposure to UV light from the sun; this is referred to as photo-aging. You may have noticed in older people that the quality of the skin over areas such as the buttocks or lower back, which are infrequently exposed to sunlight, is in better condition than skin covering the face, neck and backs of the hands. UV exposure probably causes the formation of cross-bonding between individual strands of collagen; this will result in tangled dermal collagen, contributing to wrinkles. A secondary factor in skin-related ageing is probably quality of diet or the presence of malnutrition.

Older skin is more prone to wrinkling and loss of elasticity. This can be partly explained by a reduction in the numbers of fibroblasts in the dermis. As these cells normally produce collagen and elastic fibres, the amount of these structural components of connective tissues will be reduced. In addition to loss of elasticity, this will result in reduced tensile strength and 'body'. These factors partly explain the formation of droopy skin such as 'bags under the eyes'. Loss of these tissue components also partly explains increasing skin thinning.

In older skin there is a flattening of the junction between the dermis and epidermis. As epidermal cells are nourished from dermal tissue fluid, the epidermis becomes relatively hypoxic and malnourished. This factor contributes to a reduction of up to 50% in keratinocyte replication rates. Partly as a result of this there is reduced production of epidermal lipids, resulting in dry skin. Flattening of the epidermal dermal junction also increases the probability of shearing and blister formation.

Slower rates of wound healing in elderly people are partly caused by an age-related reduction in dermal vascularity. Reduction in the numbers of peripheral sensory receptors reduces skin sensitivity. Melanocyte populations are reduced by 10–20% in older people with a resulting sensitivity to sunlight. Another obvious age related change is in hair distribution. There may be a thinning of scalp hair in men and women. Men tend to grow thicker hair on their eyebrow and ears and from their noses. Women start to grow hair above the upper lip and face.

Never mind – we all grow old unless we die first. Perhaps the key is to accept age related changes with dignity.

CHAPTER 11

Thermoregulation

Body temperature must be finely controlled. As discussed in Chapter 1, cellular biochemistry is essential for life. All intracellular biochemistry is catalysed by enzymes. These enzymes only work within narrow ranges of temperature; if the body becomes too hot or too cold enzymic function will be reduced and ultimately death will occur. Humans are biologically classified as homoiothermes because we maintain a constant body temperature. In order to achieve this balance the body needs to have mechanisms for heat gain and loss.

Heat gain

Metabolic gain

Heat is gained by the body as a result of metabolic processes. All energy chains end as heat, so whenever fuels are used heat will be generated. Increased metabolic activity in an organ will result in more heat being produced. Because the liver is a large, metabolically active organ it produces a lot of heat. Skeletal muscles also produce a lot when actively contracting. When people die they are no longer carrying out metabolic processes so body temperature drops until it is the same as the surrounding environment.

Rate of heat generation is determined by the metabolic rate of the body. This does vary between individuals and may partly explain why some people are more tolerant of cold or heat than others. Levels of thyroid hormone are a major determinant of metabolic rate.

Gain from the environment

Heat may be gained from warm environments or from infra-red radiation, emitted by the sun or other hot objects. Hot food and drink may also result in limited heat gain in the body.

Heat retention

Most of the body is insulated by a layer of subcutaneous adipose tissue; this is an excellent insulator of heat, and the thicker it is, the more it will retain heat within the body. People with a thinner adipose layer lose heat more rapidly.

Overall body mass is another factor in heat retention. When body mass is large, there will be less surface area compared to volume in comparison to a smaller person. This is called the surface area to volume ratio. In children, the surface area to volume ration is high, so they can lose heat to the environment much more quickly than adults.

Heat loss

Heat may be lost via a combination of three physical processes.

Conduction

In conduction, heat passes from warm objects to cold ones via direct contact. This explains why people can become hypothermic very quickly when immersed in cold water. Because water is in direct contact with the body, heat will pass directly from the body into the water. Conduction works particularly efficiently in the case of water because it is a good conductor of heat.

One reason we wear clothes is to keep warm. Clothes work because a layer of air is trapped near the surface of the skin. This thin layer is warmed up by the body, and because air is trapped next to the skin surface, further heat loss is prevented. Air is a particularly poor conductor of heat, so as long as we can trap some air next to the skin it will insulate us from heat loss.

Cooling due to evaporation may be considered as heat loss via conduction. When water is on the surface of the body it starts to evaporate. Evaporation describes the process of a liquid changing into a vapour. When water changes from a liquid into a vapour it requires a large amount of energy in order to do so. This energy is called the latent heat of vaporization ('latent' means 'hidden', 'vaporization' describes the process of a liquid changing into a vapour). The latent heat required is extracted from the surface of the body, which has an overall cooling effect.

Convection

Natural convection occurs when air near the surface of the body is warmed. When air is warmed the molecules of which it is made up vibrate more vigorously than they do when cold. Because they are vibrating more rapidly they take up more space when warm than they do when cold. The result of this is that the density of warm air is less than cold air. (This principle is most clearly seen in a hot air balloon where warm air provides lift.) Warm air near the surface therefore rises away from the body to be replaced by more dense, colder air from below.

Heat loss due to wind chill may be considered as forced convection. In a wind, air that has been warmed by the body, near the surface, will be blown away and replaced by cold air. More heat will then be conducted out of the body to warm up this new cold air.

Radiation

All hot objects radiate heat, mostly in the form of infra-red. Heat is therefore transferred away from the body in the form of radiation. Human skin is a fairly efficient emitter of radiation, resulting in heat loss from the body surface. Quantities of heat lost in this way are essentially the same for all skin colours. Because our clothes also possess some heat they too emit radiation into the environment. Clothes only radiate heat away from the body as a function of their surface temperature. (The hotter an object the more heat it will radiate.) Because clothes trap air, and so insulate the body, the surface temperature of clothes is much lower than the surface temperature of the body. This means we lose less heat by radiation when we are dressed than when undressed.

In a warm sunny environment we may gain more heat from solar radiation than we lose via radiation from the body surface. In this situation total heat gain will be less if we wear a covering layer over the skin. This is why clothes can also help to keep us cool in very sunny conditions.

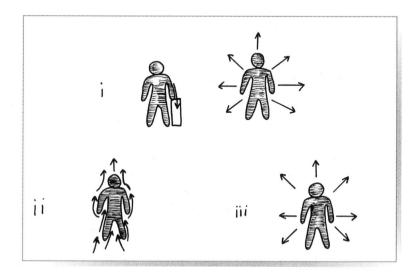

Diagram 11.1 Physical processes resulting in heat loss from the body. Arrows indicate direction of heat flow.
(i) Conduction, including heat lost by direct contact and as a result of evaporation.
(ii) Convection.
(iii) Radiation.

Body temperature

Normal body temperature varies a little between individuals. Mine is normally about 36.4°C; however, up to 37°C is considered normal. Some individuals may have temperatures which are normal for them from as low as 36°C to as high as 37.5°C. But individuals with persistently high body temperatures are uncommon; on the vast majority of times you record a temperature of 37.5°C it will be an indication of an infection or tissue damage. If the environment is very cold then core temperature may start to drop. People are particularly prone to lowering their body temperature if they are wet as well as cold. If the core temperature drops below 35°C this may be described as hypothermia.

During exercise body temperature may rise to 38°C, and vigorous exercise may elevate this as high as 40°C. However, these rises soon trigger cooling responses from such mechanisms as sweating. Whenever total heat gain exceeds heat loss, body temperature will start to rise. This can occur in very hot environments or when cooling mechanisms are unable to function. For example, soldiers have become hyperthermic while exercising in full kit on hot days. Wearing a lot of clothes prevents heat loss to the environment and reduces the evaporation of sweat. Like hypothermia, hyperthermia is a life-threatening condition.

Core temperature

This is the temperature of the body core, in the main organs. Core temperature remains relatively constant over long periods of time, although it usually varies slightly through a 24-hour period. It is normally about 0.5°C below normal early in the morning and as much as 1°C higher in the evenings. When the environment is cool or warm, core temperature will remain constant as a result of various homeostatic mechanisms discussed shortly. In ovulating women, temperature may drop slightly for about 24 hours after ovulation. Typically, temperatures are about 0.5°C higher during the second half of the menstrual cycle. These changes are not accurate enough to use as a guide to contraception but may be used to aid conception.

Peripheral temperature

Temperature on the surface of the skin or in the hands and feet may be well below core temperature, especially in cold environments. This is normal. Arms and legs have a large surface area in comparison to their volume, so have the potential to lose a lot of heat. This is useful in warm environments to increase heat loss. These factors explain why considerable proportions of the arms and legs are at or near core temperatures in hot environments, but well below in cold conditions.

Temperature detection

Thermoreceptors located in the dermis send messages to the brain that give us our sensory awareness of temperature. This is the main determinant of how hot, cold or comfortable we feel. Humans are not very tolerant of temperature change; we start to feel cold or hot with only a few degrees of ambient temperature change. 'Ambient' refers to conditions in the immediate environment. A comfortable skin temperature is usually about 33°C.

Core temperature is actually detected in the hypothalamus. An area of hypothalamus compares the temperature of the blood passing through with a set level. Neurones in the hypothalamus seem to know what this set body temperature should be. If blood temperature drops below this level, the hypothalamus initiates homeostatic mechanisms to increase body temperature. When blood temperature rises, it initiates mechanisms to lower body temperature. The hypothalamus has often been likened to a thermostat or a pair of scales.

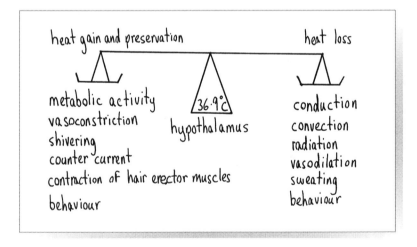

Diagram 11.2 Diagrammatic representation of the function of the hypothalamus, which maintains a balance between heat gain and loss to maintain thermal homeostasis.

When core temperature rises

This situation initiates body cooling mechanisms.

Behavioural change

When too hot, people tend to become lethargic and inactive; this will reduce heat gain from metabolism. We also go into the shade, which reduces gains from external radiation. We may choose to stand in a cooling breeze, or arrange to be fanned, if either is available. During sleep, warm people naturally adopt a 'spread out' posture to maximize surface area over which heat can be lost by radiation and convection. Increasing and decreasing clothing is an option usually available.

Peripheral vasodilation

When body temperature rises the hypothalamus causes peripheral pre-capillary sphincters to relax. This allows dilation of the arterioles, resulting in increased blood flow to the capillaries. Warm blood flowing near the surface of the body will lose heat to the environment by conduction and convection as long as air temperature is below body temperature.

Increase in blood temperature also causes a superficial peripheral venodilation (widening of the lumen of veins) in the arms and legs. Blood therefore returns to the heart via superficial peripheral veins, near the skin surface, allowing more time for heat loss to the environment.

Sweating

This is a very efficient cooling mechanism. Water deposited on the body surface extracts the latent heat of vaporization in order to evaporate. Even in very hot environments people can usually maintain normal body temperature as long as they have plenty of water to drink. This will allow them to continue producing sweat. If a person in a hot environment becomes dehydrated and can no longer sweat freely they may rapidly become hyperthermic. Dehydration may develop rapidly in hot conditions as sweating can result in fluid losses as high as 1 litre per hour.

Ambient humidity is another factor in how efficiently sweating works. In low humidity sweat will evaporate quickly, resulting in a rapid cooling effect. In humid environments, however, sweat will not evaporate efficiently. This will result in sweat remaining on the body surface without evaporating. As evaporation has not occurred, no latent heat of vaporization will be extracted, so cooling will not occur.

Hyperthermia

Cooling mechanisms only work within a limited range. If the environment continues to get hotter, or heat loss mechanisms are inhibited, then body temperature will start to rise and hyperthermia will develop. Any temperature above normal is technically a hyperthermia; however, this is not usually a major problem up to about 40°C. At temperatures above this level, the brain has a reducing capacity to function normally and the individual will progressively lose the ability to think in a coherent way. If the body temperature rises above 41°C the condition should be urgently treated. Death from hyperthermia normally occurs at about 45°C. This is because essential intracellular enzymes denature and no longer function. Denaturing means enzymes change their physical shape and so are no longer able to catalyse essential biochemistry.

When core temperature falls

This situation initiates body-warming mechanisms.

Behavioural change

When too cold, we often try to warm up by a voluntary increase in metabolic activity, waving our arms or jogging on the spot. We try to avoid further cooling from wind chill by avoiding moving air currents. Cold sleeping people naturally curl up to reduce the surface area available over which heat loss from convection and radiation may occur. We put on more clothes and seek out warm environments.

Shivering

This is rapid involuntary contraction of skeletal muscles, mostly of the upper half of the body. It is initiated and controlled by the hypothalamus. Shivering can triple metabolic rate and therefore is an effective means of thermogenesis. 'Thermogenesis' literally means 'the beginning of heat'.

Metabolic thermogenesis

Hypothermia is a particular risk in the newborn. In cold environments newborn babies should be quickly dried and wrapped up next to the mother's body. However, neonates also contain their own emergency heat generating mechanism. In various areas of the body there is brown fat, or brown adipose tissue. This is able to rapidly metabolize fatty acids to generate heat. There is debate as to how long this metabolic heating mechanism remains active, but it may well persist into childhood and even beyond.

There is evidence that people who live in cold environments for prolonged periods increase basal metabolic rate by increasing thyroxine levels. This mechanism probably takes several weeks to develop and is associated with an increased size of the thyroid gland. Metabolic rates, and therefore thermogenesis, in people exposed to cold for several weeks are increased. Artic explorers lose a large percentage of body fat over a few months, presumably because the fat has been burned up to support the increased metabolic rate.

Arterial vasoconstriction

In order to preserve heat in the physiologically essential core organs, blood supply to the cold peripheries such as hands and feet is reduced. Arterial supply of blood is restricted by reduction of arterial lumens. This is why we get cold hands and feet in cold environments.

When the body is cold, it is essential to minimize heat loss through the skin. This can be done by reducing skin temperature. Precapillary sphincters in the arterioles supplying blood to dermal capillary beds contract when it is cold. This results in peripheral vasoconstriction, greatly reducing the perfusion of the skin. Blood that would normally perfuse the capillaries is transferred directly from small arteries to small veins via shunt vessels. Reduction of superficial blood flow explains why cold people look pale.

If people are injured in cold conditions, vasoconstrictive mechanisms can help to reduce blood loss. This is why people with external haemorrhage should not be warmed up, until they are in a situation

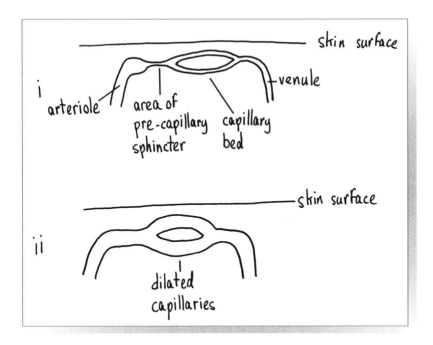

Diagram 11.3 Body temperature is partly regulated
by varying the perfusion of superficial capillaries.
(i)   When the body is too cold, pre-capillary
      sphincters constrict reducing the volumes of
      warm blood flowing near the body surface.
(ii) When the body is too hot, pre-capillary
      sphincters dilate increasing the volumes of
      warm blood flowing near the body surface.

where the bleeding vessels can be ligated. Conversely, if part of the
body is warm and well perfused, bleeding may be more severe than it
would be in a cooler environment.

In humans, reduction of arterial blood supply to cold extremities
is a very efficient mechanism. Reduction in blood supply can be so
pronounced that the temperature in extremities may drop to 0°C.
When this happens the tissue freezes. As a tissue freezes, ice crystals
form in the cytosol of the cells. As ice forms in the cells it expands,
and this results in rupture of cell membranes, disrupting tissue integrity
at the cellular level. Tissue necrosis (necrosis means death) caused by
this freezing mechanism is called frostbite and often necessitates

amputations. Interestingly, this process of tissue destruction on freezing explains why people who are frozen after death – in the hope of being brought back to life in the future – never will be.

Venoconstriction

In order to conserve heat, superficial veins also constrict. This obliges blood returning from the periphery to return to the heart via the deep venous systems of the legs and arms. As warm blood is kept away from the cold surface, less heat will be lost from the skin surface.

Venoconstriction of peripheral veins also preserves heat via a second mechanism. Deep veins often run close to arteries. This closeness allows for a counter-current heat exchange mechanism to operate. Counter-current systems operate when two fluids flow near each other in opposite directions. Remember, in conduction, heat always passes from hot areas

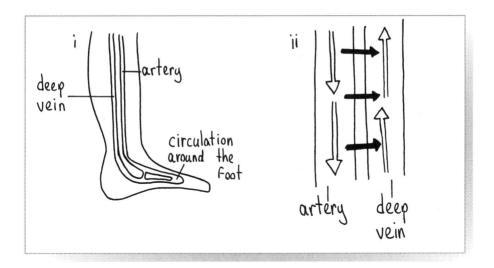

Diagram 11.4

(i) Anatomical arrangement of deep blood vessels which facilitates counter-current heat exchange between an artery and a vein.

(ii) Close-up view of an artery and a deep vein. White arrows indicate the direction of blood flow and dark arrows indicate heat transfer.

to cold ones. As warm arterial blood passes down the limb, heat is directly transferred to the cooler venous blood. This means returning venous blood is warmed and the arterial blood cooled. Blood entering a cold extremity is therefore already cooled while blood returning to the warm core is already warmed. This allows cold peripheries to remain perfused and oxygenated without losing additional heat from the blood.

Contraction of hair erector muscles

Contraction of these muscles causes the hair to 'stand on end'. This will increase the thickness of the boundary layer of insulating air, increasing the insulation of the body, so conserving heat.

Hypothermia

Heat gain and conservation mechanisms only work within a limited range. If the environment continues to get colder, or heat gain mechanisms are inhibited, then body temperature will start to fall and hypothermia will develop. When a person becomes hypothermic, their metabolic rate will suffer a corresponding drop. At a temperature of 27°C the metabolic rate is 2.5 times lower than at 37°C. Therefore any reduction in body temperature will reduce metabolic heat gain, and so lower body temperature further. The drop in body temperature will cause a further drop in metabolic rate, setting up a downward spiral leading to death from hypothermia.

If you are ever in a situation where hypothermia is a possibility, it is important not to go to sleep, as this will allow the vicious downward spiral to start. If you keep awake you can generate heat by voluntary muscular activity and so maintain metabolic rate and core temperature. Sleep is a particular temptation in developing hypothermia because the lowered temperature reduces the metabolic activity of the brain, which makes us feel sleepy. People who have been rescued from hypothermic coma report that apart from feeling cold for a time they just felt drowsy and went to sleep. This would seem to indicate that death from hypothermia is not too unpleasant.

Because living hypothermic patients may be comatose and cold they may appear to be dead. In cases where death is suspected in hypothermia the patient should be warmed up before death is pronounced. Sometimes when patients are warmed up they recover. There is a reliable saying in Accident and Emergency practice – 'No one is dead until they are warm and dead.' In other words, only pronounce death once you have returned body temperature to normal.

Alcohol

Apparently an order of Swiss monks used to send St Bernard dogs to the aid of people trapped in snowdrifts. Around their necks were tied small barrels of brandy.

When cold people drink alcohol they feel warmer. This is because alcohol is a peripheral vasodilator so increases dermal capillary blood flow. Warm blood stimulates dermal warm thermoreceptors; however, excessive amounts of heat are lost to the cold environment at the same time. Alcohol therefore reverses the natural vasoconstrictive response to cold. Most of the unfortunate people supplied with brandy by the well-meaning monks and their dogs would therefore rapidly become hypothermic and die.

Fever

Infections are often caused by bacteria or viruses. Various foreign substances released from these infectious agents enter the blood and are collectively referred to as pyrogens. A pyrogen initiates a pyrexia or fever. It seems the thermoregulatory centre of the hypothalamus is designed to detect the presence of pyrogens. When detected the hypothalamus increases the 'set point' for body temperature. Initially, the body temperature will be normal but the person will feel cold. Heat generating and conserving measures will be initiated, resulting in an increase in body temperature. The reason the hypothalamus increases body temperature is to optimize the function of the immune system which works best at an increased temperature, probably about 39°C. Once the infection has been overcome, cooling mechanisms will return body temperature to normal. It therefore seems that pyrexia is a normal protective response to infection and perhaps we should be less hasty in our use of antipyretics in older children and adults.

Young children are unable to effectively regulate their body temperature. If a fever is developing in children it could rise to dangerous levels very quickly. Pyrexia in children can cause febrile convulsions.

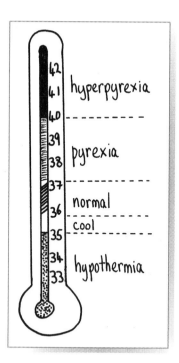

Diagram 11.5 A guide to the classification of body temperature in the clinical setting.

In order to reduce this risk it is normal to treat pyrexia in children at a fairly early stage. The peak age for febrile convulsions is between 5 months and 6 years old.

Pyrexia may also be caused by tissue damage in the absence of infection; this may be seen after an infarction when the blood supply to part of the body is occluded. You may also see this effect after trauma or surgery.

CHAPTER 12

The liver

The liver is the largest gland in the body; in fact, it is the largest solid organ, and only the skin has a greater total mass. It is accurate to classify the liver as an exocrine gland as it produces approximately 500 ml of bile per day. In addition to the production of bile, the liver is involved in many of the biochemical processes that are necessary within the body. This is why the liver is sometimes referred to as the 'chemical factory' of the body.

Blood supply

Unusually, the liver receives about 70% of its blood supply from the hepatic portal vein (HPV), which drains blood directly from the gastrointestinal tract (see page 98). However, in order to support metabolism, liver cells also need a supply of oxygen, which is supplied via the hepatic artery. After circulating through the liver, venous blood is drained into the inferior vena cava via three hepatic veins. Be careful not to mix up the hepatic portal vein and the hepatic vein in your mind. The HPV carries blood to the liver from the gut; the hepatic vein drains blood from the liver, back into the systemic venous return.

Structure related to function

Position

The liver occupies most of the upper right quadrant of the abdominal cavity. Rounded upper surfaces fit snugly under the domed diaphragm

Diagram 12.1 Diagrammatic representation of the flow of blood to and from the liver; the flow of bile to the duodenum is also indicated.

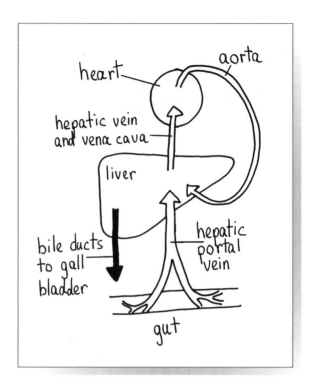

while the lower surfaces are fairly sharp, giving a wedge-shaped appearance from the side. In young children the relatively large size of the liver explains why their upper abdomens protrude.

Lobes

The liver is composed of four lobes. However, from the front only two lobes are visible; these are simply called the right and left lobe, the right being significantly larger. From the back two additional smaller lobes can be distinguished, called the quadrate and caudate lobes.

Lobules

Within the lobes of the liver are numerous lobules, separated from each other by connective tissue. Lobules are usually five- or six-sided and are cylindrical. At the corners of the lobules are branches of the HPV, hepatic artery and bile ducts; collectively these three vessels are

Diagram 12.2 A section of liver made up of lobules.

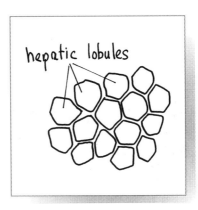

hepatic lobules

referred to as a triad. A normal liver contains from 50 000 to 100 000 lobule units, which vary in diameter from 0.8 to 2 mm.

Lobules are the functional units of the liver. Individual liver cells are called hepatocytes. In an individual lobule, hepatocytes are arranged around a central vein, like spokes around a hub in a wheel. It is a radial arrangement of cells. Typically the hepatocytes are arranged in a row, two cells thick. These two rows of cells are described as a hepatic cellular plate. Between pairs of hepatic cellular plates are the blood sinusoids. A sinusoid is essentially a type of blood capillary with very porous walls, allowing more contact that usual between the blood and tissue cells. I often just think of these sinusoids as hepatic capillaries.

Sinusoids receive blood from two sources: first, from a branch of the hepatic portal vein, and second, from a branch of the hepatic artery. Again this is unusual; venous and arterial blood mix in the sinusoids as they pass through the lobule. This arrangement supplies hepatocytes with nutrient-rich blood from the hepatic portal vein and oxygenated blood from the hepatic artery. Cells lining the sinusoid are able to selectively absorb substances from the blood, carry out chemical processes, and then secrete the products back into the blood of the same sinusoid.

Liver sinusoids also contain macrophages called Kupffer cells in their walls. These phagocytes break down old red blood cells and protect the liver against the possibility of infection.

In the centre of each lobule are small tributaries of the hepatic vein. Blood from the sinusoids drains directly into this central lobular vein. This joins up with other lobular veins that eventually become one of the three large hepatic veins.

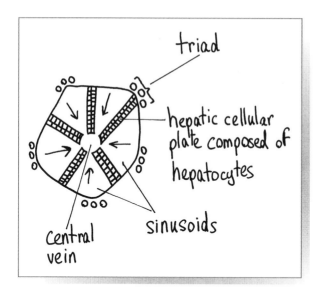

Diagram 12.3 Simplified view of the radial arrangement of hepatocytes and sinusoids in a liver lobule. Arrows indicate direction of blood flow through the lobule.

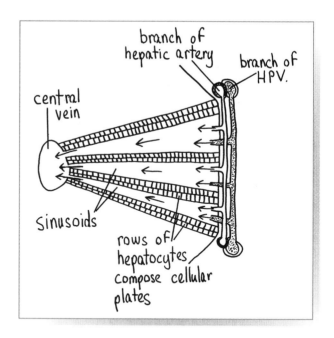

Diagram 12.4 Simplified view of a 'slice' of a lobule. Blood enters from small branches of the HPV and hepatic artery. Arrows indicate direction of blood flow (bile drainage vessels are not shown).

Between the two rows of hepatocytes are microscopic channels called canaliculi. Individual hepatocytes produce bile, which they excrete from the cell into these canaliculi. These in turn drain into the small bile channels of the triads, which are tributaries of larger hepatic bile ducts. This arrangement means that bile flow in canaliculi is in the opposite direction to the blood passing through the sinusoids. The separation of the sinusoids (blood channels) and canaliculi (bile

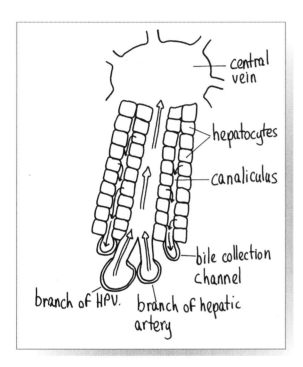

Diagram 12.5 Cross-section of part of a liver lobule. This shows two hepatic cellular plates with blood flowing through the sinusoid between. Individual hepatocytes excrete bile into the canaliculi which then flows between the two rows of cells to be collected in a small bile duct. The three vessels of the triad are running in and out of the plane of the page. White arrows indicate blood flow and dark arrows bile flow.

Diagram 12.6 Transverse section of the two rows of cells which form a hepatic cellular plate. The canaliculus is actually formed between the two rows of cells. Bile produced in the individual hepatocytes is only excreted into the canaliculi. This means bile is only excreted from one side of the hepatocytes as the other side is in contact with the blood. Arrows indicate direction of bile flow.

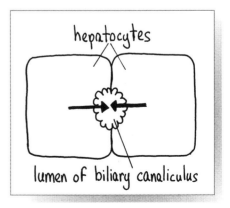

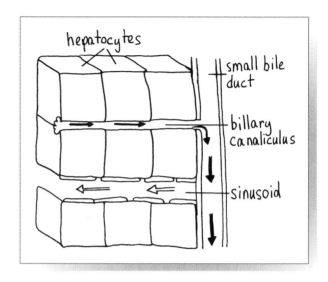

channels) prevents bile and blood mixing. Bile flows into progressively larger bile ducts that eventually unite to form the right and left hepatic duct and then the common hepatic duct.

Bile

Bile is alkaline, with a pH of about 8; it is largely water but also contains bile salts and bile pigments.

Bile salts are important in the physical emulsification of fats in the digestive process. They are produced from cholesterol, in the individual hepatocytes, and secreted into the bile. Sodium chloride and bicarbonate are also incorporated into bile.

Bilirubin is the principle bile pigment. When red blood cells reach the end of their life they are broken down by macrophages, mostly located in the spleen. Macrophages in the liver itself also break down some old red blood cells. When the haemoglobin molecules are broken down, a yellow pigment called bilirubin is left over. This bilirubin is extracted from the blood by liver cells. In the cells, bilirubin is joined on to another molecule called glucuronic acid. This process is called conjugation, which just means to 'join together'. Conjugation increases the solubility of bilirubin so it may be carried in solution in bile. Although it is true that bilirubin is essentially an excretory product, bile pigments do colour and partly deodorize faeces.

If the liver is unable to excrete bile, bilirubin will dam back into the liver and ultimately into the blood. This can be seen in the whites of the eyes initially and later, if the condition becomes more severe, in the skin. This yellow discoloration is called jaundice.

Liver functions

In addition to the production of bile, the liver is involved in a wide range of physiological processes.

Carbohydrate metabolism

The liver is important in the maintenance of blood sugar concentrations. Excess glucose in the blood is absorbed by the liver and converted into glycogen. This is stored, then when blood sugar levels are low it is converted back into glucose and released. Liver cells are also able to convert amino acids into glucose when there is a shortage in the blood. The liver can also convert galactose and fructose (two other small sugar molecules) into glucose. Maintenance of blood glucose levels is essential as the brain must have a constant supply of glucose to fuel its metabolic activity. If there is no glucose at all in the blood, brain function will cease.

Fat metabolism

Liver cells are able to process one type of fat into another type that may be needed in various areas of the body. For example, some types of fat are needed for the production of cell membranes and organelles, as well as numerous biochemical processes throughout the body. In addition, excess protein and carbohydrate is converted into fat for storage. This is why eating too much carbohydrate or protein also causes us to put on weight.

If there is alcohol in the blood hepatocytes are able to absorb fat for processing as normal. However, alcohol prevents the liver cells from secreting fat. This means that if there is alcohol in the blood every day, liver cells will start to accumulate fat. The increased amounts of fat in the liver cells causes the liver to become fatty and bulky. If this is prolonged, liver cells will start to die and be replaced by fibrous tissue; this is called cirrhosis. If a person stops drinking while the liver is still at the fatty stage the condition is reversible; however, once cirrhosis has developed the liver damage is irreversible.

Protein metabolism

The liver carries out numerous biochemical processes on amino acids and proteins. Before proteins can be used to produce carbohydrates or fat they must first be chemically broken down. This breakdown of amino acids is called deamination and occurs almost exclusively in the hepatocytes.

Proteins are composed largely of carbon, hydrogen, oxygen and nitrogen. Fats and carbohydrates contain only carbon, hydrogen and oxygen. This means that when proteins are broken down, nitrogen is left over as a waste product. Nitrogen in solution forms toxic ammonia, and this must be rapidly removed from the blood. Additional ammonia, produced by bacteria, is absorbed from the gut. In liver failure waste ammonia is not continuously removed so it accumulates in the blood. This causes a condition referred to as hepatic coma, which leads to death. Hepatocytes take up ammonia and chemically convert it into a much less toxic, highly soluble, nitrogen-containing substance called urea. This is removed from the blood by the kidneys and excreted in urine.

Liver cells are able to change the form of some amino acids. Human proteins contain 20 different amino acids, so these need to be available for the processes of growth and repair. Of these 20 amino acids, 10 can be produced in the liver from other amino acids, but the other 10 cannot be converted. Therefore, the 10 that cannot be converted from others must be present in the diet if health is to be maintained. These 10 that cannot be produced in the liver are referred to as essential amino acids, because they must be part of the diet. Amino acids which can be produced in the liver by conversion are called non-essential, not because they are not necessary for normal physiology but because health may be maintained even if they are not part of the diet. The process of converting one amino acid to another is called transamination.

The liver also forms all of the plasma proteins except the immune globulins. Albumin is produced by hepatocytes and released into the blood. This plasma protein is essential to maintain the osmolarity of the plasma, which is needed to facilitate osmotic reabsorption of tissue fluids. Albumin also acts as a 'carrier' molecule, transporting some substances around the circulatory system. Some drugs are also transported bound to albumin.

Liver cells also produce several of the clotting factors such as prothrombin and fibrinogen. If liver function is compromised, production of these plasma proteins is reduced; this rapidly leads to haemorrhagic problems as the patients are no longer able to form blood clots. Angiotensinogen is also a short protein molecule produced by the liver cells.

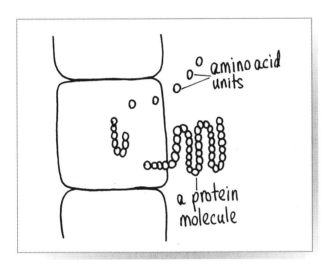

Diagram 12.8 This diagram illustrates the function of the individual hepatocyte using protein synthesis as an example. Individual amino acids are absorbed from the blood flowing through the sinusoid. In the cell the amino acids are chemically combined to produce a protein molecule which is then secreted back into the blood flowing through the sinusoid.

Storage of nutrients

The liver stores the fat-soluble vitamins A, D, E and K; it also holds reserves of vitamin B_{12}. These reserves may be extensive; enough vitamin A is stored to supply the body for 10 months with no dietary intake. Sufficient B_{12} is stored to prevent deficiency developing for several years. Iron is also stored in the liver cells in the form of a molecule called ferritin.

Breakdown of toxins and drugs

Liver cells are capable of recognizing and chemically breaking down a wide range of toxins. Bacterial activity in the gut generates large amounts of toxins that are transported to the liver by the HPV. These are broken down to less toxic substances that may be excreted by the kidneys or incorporated into bile for excretion in the faeces.

Most drugs are recognized as 'toxins' by the liver and are broken down to metabolites. In the liver cells many drugs are oxidized or conjugated to increase their solubility in water. These processes are facilitated by numerous hepatic enzymes, the best known of these being the cytochrome P450 group. (You will certainly come across these if you study pharmacology.) Once the drug metabolites (breakdown products) are soluble they are usually excreted readily in the urine, although a few drug metabolites are excreted in bile. If there is liver failure drugs will not be broken down and can reach toxic levels.

Most hormones are also broken down by the liver after a period of time circulating in the blood. Liver failure can therefore result in increased plasma concentrations in such hormones as thyroxine, oestrogen and cortisol.

Generation of heat

As a result of ongoing metabolic processes in the liver, a lot of heat is generated. This makes an important contribution to body temperature, especially during periods of reduced muscular activity.

CHAPTER 13

Inflammation and immunity

The inflammatory response is both normal and necessary. Inflammation is the first stage in the healing process. Inflammation literally means 'to set afire'; the suffix '-itis' is used to describe an inflammatory response, e.g. tonsillitis, appendicitis, peritonitis.

Causes of inflammation

Any insult to a tissue may lead to a local inflammatory response. Although inflammation may be caused by a wide variety of tissue insults, the nature of the response is always the same.

Mechanical trauma, such as dropping a hammer on your foot, may cause inflammation. Direct tissue contact with any corrosive agents such as acids or alkalis provides another range of possible causes. For example, leakage of bile or intestinal contents into the peritoneal cavity can cause severe peritonitis. Thermal injuries, caused by exposure to excessive heat or cold, will lead to inflammation. An inflammatory response may also be caused by immunological reactions; this may well be the cause of swollen, painful joints in rheumatoid arthritis. A similar immunological reaction explains sensitivity to some environmental agents; pollen grains are an example of this, as anyone who suffers from hay fever is only too aware. The final common cause is infection: bacteria and the toxins they release stimulate an immunological inflammatory response.

Inflammatory mediators

An inflammatory response is stimulated by local release of inflammatory mediators. When a tissue is insulted there is a release of histamine from mast cells located in the tissues. Mast cells are similar to basophils, a form of leucocyte found in the blood. However, mast cells remain localized in tissues and do not circulate.

Fatty acids from damaged cell membranes are acted on by an enzyme in the tissues called cyclo-oxygenase. This converts the fatty acids into chemicals called prostaglandins. Histamine and prostaglandins both facilitate an inflammatory response.

Features of inflammation

The five clinical features of inflammation are redness, heat, swelling, pain and loss of function.

Redness and heat

Vasodilation of local blood vessels increases blood supply to the area; this is called a hyperaemia. Increased volumes of blood give the inflamed area a reddened appearance. Inflamed areas feel warmer than the surrounding body surface. This heat is also explained by the increased volumes of warm blood circulating near the surface of the body.

Swelling

Because the capillaries dilate, the physical size of the gaps in their walls increases, thus increasing their permeability. Increased capillary permeability increases the volume of tissue fluid formed and also allows larger molecules such as plasma proteins to escape into the tissues. White cells such as monocytes and neutrophils may squeeze out through the dilated capillary walls into the tissue spaces. The resultant fluid is termed inflammatory exudate. It is the presence of increased volumes of fluid in the tissues that causes the swelling.

Pain and loss of function

In addition to dilating local blood vessels, inflammatory mediators act on the pain receptors. Inflamed areas are very sensitive to touch or movement because the inflammatory mediators increase the sensitivity of local nociceptors. They do this by reducing the depolarization threshold, making it more likely a stimulus will produce a new nerve

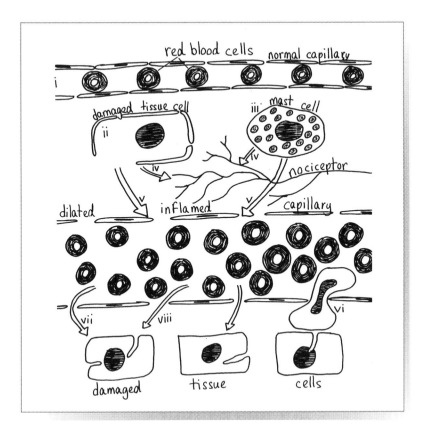

Diagram 13.1 The process of inflammation.

(i)   A normal capillary has a narrow lumen and relatively tight junctions between the endothelial cells that comprise the wall. Red cells pass along the small capillaries one at a time.

(ii) Damaged tissue cells release fatty acids which are converted into prostaglandins; these act as inflammatory mediators.

(iii) Mast cells release histamine, another inflammatory mediator.

(iv) Inflammatory mediators sensitize local nociceptors producing hyperalgesia; this will also lead to 'guarding' of the injured or infected area.

(v)   Inflammatory mediators cause dilation of local blood vessels leading to hyperaemia; this will increase the oxygenation of the area.

(vi) White blood cells are able to migrate through the dilated capillary wall; once in the tissue spaces they will phagocytose dead tissue cells and bacteria.

(vii) Increased supplies of tissue fluid move out of the blood into the tissue spaces – transporting amino acids, vitamins and minerals. These building blocks are necessary for regeneration of the damaged tissue.

(viii)Fibrinogen is able to escape from the dilated capillary to form physical barriers which will aid in the consolidation of infection. Immune proteins also migrate out into the tissue spaces.

impulse. Even the pulse in a tissue may be a sufficient stimulus to cause pain. You may remember your thumb throbbing the last time you hit it with a hammer. This increased pain response is termed a hyperalgesia.

The purpose of inflammation

Wound healing is a metabolically active process. This is because damaged areas need to be repaired and new tissues constructed. Both of these processes are anabolic (they involve building up new large molecules), and energy is always required for building work. A hyperaemia fuels this requirement by increasing the blood supply to the area and thereby delivering extra glucose and oxygen.

Increase in the volumes of tissue fluid increases the supply of amino acids, vitamins and minerals to the damaged area. Amino acids are essential to build up new proteins, and vitamins help to catalyse some of these anabolic reactions. Several minerals, such as zinc, are also necessary for normal healing.

Increased capillary permeability will allow fibrinogen (a blood clotting protein) to enter the tissues. In the tissue spaces, fibrinogen is converted into strands of insoluble fibrin. This forms a provisional structural framework for the new tissue and allows the passage of cells required for further healing. Fibrin also forms a physical mesh that helps to isolate areas of infection; this promotes consolidation (isolating infection together in one place) and inhibits spread of any infection.

Immunoglobulins are antibodies or immune proteins. These pass from blood into the tissue spaces through the dilated capillary walls, and can quickly start to combat any infection that might have been introduced into an injury.

White blood cells are able to escape into the tissues where they phagocytose dead tissue cells and bacteria. Removal of dead tissue is essential to allow young cells to migrate over living tissues. Living cells will not travel over areas of dead tissue. Also, if dead tissue is left in a wound it acts as a ready-formed habitat and food source for potential infection. Leucocytes also release chemical mediators that promote the healing process. Maggots introduced on to a wound also preferentially eat dead (necrotic) tissue. In this sense their debridement role is similar to that of phagocytes ('debride' means to remove foreign or dead material from a wound). This is the basis of the revival of the ancient treatment of larval therapy.

Immobilization of an injured area promotes healing. When an area is injured and painful, local muscles are stimulated to contract and protect the injury. For example, if you sprain an ankle the lower leg muscles will tighten to 'splint' the injured area. This reaction is referred to as muscle 'guarding'.

From these examples it can be seen why inflammation is essential for normal healing. This is illustrated by the poor wound healing observed in patients taking corticosteroid drugs that inhibit the inflammatory response.

The spectre of infectious disease

There has recently been an increased awareness of the problem posed by infectious diseases with the emergence of antibiotic-resistant bacteria. However, we live in a world full of micro-organisms and some of these have the potential to cause disease.

Throughout human history infectious disease has been a constant threat. The Bible describes the plague of Ashod; this occurred in what is the modern day Gaza Strip around 1100 BC, probably killing many thousands of people. The Black Death arose in fourteenth-century England and killed an estimated 100 000 people. Bubonic plague in 1665 killed at least 68 000 people in London alone. Cholera epidemics in England during the 1850s also killed thousands of people. Between 1568 and 1620 the indigenous population of Mexico fell from 30 million to 1.6 million, largely due to infectious disease introduced by European invaders to which the local people had no immunity. Influenza killed between 20 to 40 million people in 1919; it is likely that such a pandemic will strike us again. Smallpox killed 300 million people in the twentieth century before it was eradicated. In many developing countries, 70–80% of deaths are caused by infections. Children under five are often extensively affected; diarrhoea and vomiting is still the most common cause of death in the world's children, killing many millions each year. Three million children die from malaria in Africa every year.

Any micro-organism with the potential to cause disease is a pathogenic micro-organism. (In clinical practice this is often abbreviated to 'pathogen' or 'bug', referred to in common speech as a germ.

Micro-organism is usually abbreviated to microbe.) Even bacteria that do not normally cause disease, such as those in the colon, certainly cause problems if they get into the blood, peritoneum or bladder. The common forms of organisms that may cause disease are bacteria, viruses, fungi, protozoa and parasitic worms. Infection simply means the presence of a microbe in a body tissue or structure.

Fortunately, humans are equipped with a wide range of mechanisms to protect us against this ever-present threat. Immunity may be described as the ability of the body to resist infections. Normally the body tissues are sterile, completely free of any microbes at all.

Two types of immunity

The body is protected against micro-organisms in basically two ways. The first is by innate immunity; this is also referred to as non-specific. These mechanisms act against a wide range of potential infectious agents in a non-discriminating way. Secondly, immunity may be acquired, also called specific or adaptive immunity. In this form of immunity the body learns how to combat a particular species of micro-organism.

Leucocytes

White cells are essential for innate and adaptive immunity. Although they are often called white blood cells, some are found in the tissues as well. All of the leucocytes derive from stem cells found in the bone marrow. It is useful to consider the leucocytes as cells involved in innate and adaptive immunity separately, although in reality the boundaries are blurred and there are interactions between the two groups.

Innate immunity

The structures and mechanisms of innate immunity already exist in the body before there is any contact with a particular potential infection. In innate immunity there is no change in the structure or mechanism involved as a result of exposure to a potential infection.

Skin

Skin is a barrier to nearly all potential pathogens as long as it remains intact. However, when the skin is broken, the way is clear for organisms from the exterior to enter. This simple principle explains why wounds may become infected. Keratin in the outer layers of the epidermis improves the hardness and quality of the physical barrier. Oily sebum prevents skin from drying out. Dry, cracked skin is much more likely to become infected than oily skin. Sweat also contains acids that kill bacteria.

Mucous membranes

Mucous membranes, lined with mucus, are able to prevent the transmission of most potential pathogens as long as the surface remains intact. Such mucous membrane is found in the mouth, inside the eyelids and lining male and female genital tracts. Some organisms such as those that cause sexually transmitted disease (STD) are able to penetrate intact mucous membranes. Human immunodeficiency virus (HIV) can pass through intact membranes, but not readily. Perhaps one of the reasons HIV spread so quickly through many African countries was because there was already a lot of pre-existing STD in the population. This would have disrupted the integrity of the genital mucous membranes, leaving, in effect, an open door through which the HIV could get in and infect the individual.

Tears and saliva

Mucus, tears and saliva all contain lysozyme. This is an enzyme that does not act against human tissues but will digest bacterial cell walls. The presence of lysozyme helps to keep these areas free from infection for most of the time, despite being always exposed to the outside world.

Respiratory system defences

The respiratory system is protected by hairs and mucus in the nose. Much of the mucous membrane lining the respiratory tract is also covered with cilia. Bacteria stick to mucus, which is then wafted into the trachea by the beating action of cilia. Coughing and sneezing bring up the mucus containing the trapped bacteria into the oropharynx. General mobility and change of respiratory patterns aids this expectoration of sputum. Patients on bed rest are at increased risk of sputum stasis and subsequent infection, which may lead on to bronchopneumonia.

Acid in the stomach

Hydrochloric acid in the stomach kills most organisms that are swallowed in food. Some elderly people produce less stomach acid than they used to, increasing their risk of infective gastritis. The alkaline nature of the small intestine is also active against some organisms.

Competition from harmless organisms

Areas of the body such as the colon, mouth and vagina contain large numbers of bacteria. This situation is normal; the bacteria compose the normal 'flora'. The presence of flora means that there is competition from harmless bacteria if any harmful organisms attempt to colonize the area. This means any pathogenic organisms entering are unlikely to be established. Organisms that live with us in this symbiotic way are called commensal; by living together we benefit each other. The value of this competition to us can be seen when antibiotics kill off the normal flora in the gut and vagina, causing diarrhoea and thrush respectively. Antibiotics may also be a factor in the cause of irritable bowel syndrome where fungal infections may be part of the problem.

Flushing effects

Flushing effects occur wherever there is a flow of fluid from one place to another. Any bacteria present are moved along with the flow. Tears wash over the surface of the eye and saliva through the mouth before it is swallowed. Bile is produced in the liver and flows down the bile ducts and into the gallbladder before flowing on to the bowel.

Urine is produced in the kidneys; the one-way flow down the urinary tract washes out any bacteria that may be present. This is why it is important to drink plenty of water if there is a urinary infection; larger volumes of water will help to flush bacteria out of the body. The importance of flushing effects is clearly seen if there is an obstruction leading to stasis. For example, a bile stone may block the flow of bile leading to infection of the gallbladder; this is called cholecystitis. Obstruction to the flow of urine, or passing small volumes of urine, increases the likelihood of urinary tract infections (UTIs). Diarrhoea is another flushing mechanism.

Complement

Some body fluids and blood contain a series of about 20 proteins collectively referred to as complement. These form a cascade that may be triggered by the presence of bacterial cells. The final component of the cascade is a protein that forms the shape of a tube. This tubular protein has an exciting sounding name, membrane attack protein; it works by puncturing a hole through the outer wall and cell membrane of bacterial cells. Water from the body fluids is then free to enter the bacterial cell causing it to swell. Once a certain volume of water has entered, the cell will burst, just like an overfilled balloon. This will clearly kill the bacterial cell.

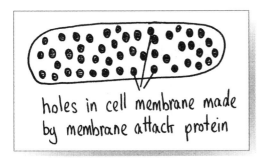

holes in cell membrane made by membrane attack protein

Diagram 13.2 The effect of membrane attack protein on an *E. coli* bacterial cell.

Interferon

When certain cells are invaded by viral particles they releases a group of chemicals called interferons. Viruses can only reproduce by hijacking a host cell. Once a new cell is infected, the virus causes it to manufacture more viral particles; it does this by taking over the host cell's normal protein synthesizing mechanisms. When the cell has produced a large number of new viruses it will burst, releasing many new viral particles into a tissue to infect more body cells.

Interferons from an infected cell will diffuse to the body cells in the surrounding area. They communicate with adjacent cells by binding to specific interferon receptor sites on the external cell membranes. When the interferon receptor is stimulated two things will happen. First, the cell will be stimulated to produce specific antiviral enzymes; these inhibit the ability of the virus to express its own genetic material, so they cannot make copies of themselves. Second, the ability of the cell to synthesize any new proteins is inhibited (interferons interfere with the cell's ability to produce proteins). If these body cells are no longer able to synthesize proteins they will not be able to produce new viruses. Interferon therefore essentially creates a barrier (a sort of 'fire break') around infected cells. Some forms of interferon also act against some cancer cells.

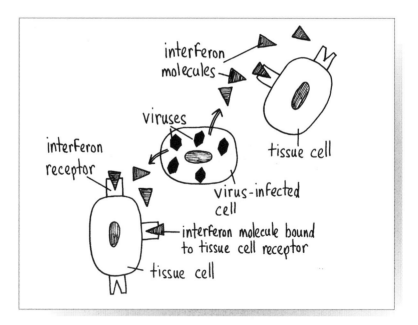

Diagram 13.3 A virus-infected cell releases interferon which combines with a specific receptor on surrounding cells. Activation of the receptor by interferon inhibits the production of viral particles, should the cell become infected. (In reality the interferon molecules and receptors are several hundred times smaller than illustrated; this is true of all of the signal molecules and receptors illustrated in this chapter.)

Opsonins

Opsonins are a form of chemical labelling system used by the immune system to clearly identify foreign material for destruction. There are a variety of chemicals which may act as opsonins including some components of the complement cascade, some antibodies and other proteins in the bloodstream. Opsonins bind onto the surface of particular components of the pathogen (antigenic molecules), which they are able to recognize as being foreign. This is possible because the chemical makeup of micro-organisms is different from the cells of the body. In addition to the ability to bind to foreign material, opsonins can also bind to receptors on the surface of phagocytes. In other words they form a bridge between antigen and phagocyte. So opsonins adhere the pathogen to the phagocyte, making its destruction

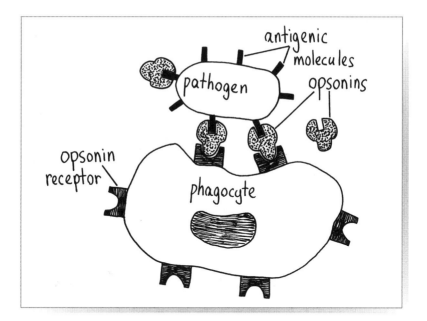

Diagram 13.4 The process of opsonization helps in the identification and adherence of an antigenic foreign organism to a phagocyte. Phagocytosis and death of the microbe will rapidly follow.

inevitable. Phagocytosis can work without opsonins but opsonization increases the efficiency of the process.

Cytotoxicity

Natural killer (NK) cells and eosinophils are able to directly kill other cells. Eosinophils come alongside foreign material and essentially bomb it. Digestive enzymes and other toxins are released from the eosinophil on to the foreign target. These damage the cell membrane of the pathogen and this is usually enough to kill the cell. This mechanism is also effective against a wide range of multicellular parasites that may invade the body. In parasitic infections the number of eosinophils is raised.

NK cells are large granular lymphocytes. They are able to act against body cells with a wide range of viral infections. NK cells are able to recognize when a body cell has become infected. When a cell has been taken over by a virus, some viral glycoproteins appear on the surface of the cell membrane; it is these viral fragments the NK cells are able to recognize. Once the NK cell has identified an infected body cell it comes alongside and releases a chemical called perforin. As its name suggests, perforin perforates the outer cell membrane of the infected cell, causing it to swell and burst. The NK cell therefore attacks the viral infection by killing infected cells. In is now widely accepted that NK cells also protect us against some forms of cancer by identifying and killing malignant cells. It is currently unclear how important this activity is in maintenance of health; however, some malignant disease may be caused by a lack of NK activity.

Cells involved in innate immunity

There are three types of white cells involved in innate immunity; these are the granulocytes, monocytes and the NKs discussed above. Granulocytes occur in three forms: neutrophils are the most common white cell type in the blood; the other two are eosinophils and basophils. Mast cells found in tissues are a form of basophil. Eosinophils also spend most of their time in the tissues. Granulocytes are named because of the granular appearance of the cytoplasm. The granules contain various substances, some of which are capable of digesting bacteria in the process of phagocytosis. While eosinophils

Diagram 13.5 Natural killer cells attack
(i) a cancer cell and
(ii) a virally infected cell.

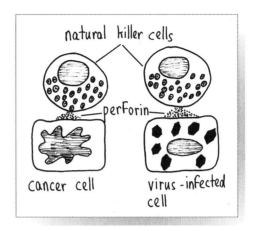

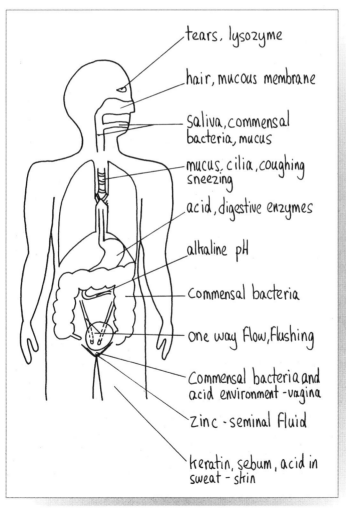

Diagram 13.6 Review of the main physical and chemical mechanisms of innate immunity.

and basophils are capable of phagocytosis, it is the neutrophils that are most active in this eating process. If we develop an infection the numbers of neutrophils in the blood increases.

Monocytes may also be found in the blood and tissues. So-called wandering monocytes circulate in the blood. These circulating cells are attracted to areas of infection or injury where they are able to migrate out of the inflamed capillaries. Once in the tissues they grow in size and are then referred to as macrophages (big eaters). Other macrophages are described as being fixed. These seem to live permanently in a particular tissue or organ. This means that if an infection gets into the organ, there is a ready-made phagocytic defence force in place. Fixed macrophages have been identified in a range of tissues including brain, lungs, liver, lymph nodes, spleen, kidneys, synovial joints and bone marrow.

Adaptive immunity

Acquired or adaptive immunity only develops after there has been contact with a particular antigen. An individual is said to be immune to a particular pathogen when it may be introduced into the body without causing illness. In contrast to innate immunity, the immune system is changed as a result of exposure to a particular antigen.

Acquired immunity is specific to a particular antigen. For example, previous exposure to the measles virus will have allowed the immune system to adapt, generating immunity to any future measles infection. However, because the response is specific, the individual may still suffer from mumps, influenza or, indeed, any other antigenic organism it has not previously been exposed to.

Antigens

An antigen is anything the immune system recognizes as being foreign. Antigens generate an immune response in the body. It is antigens that stimulate the production of antibodies, which are immune proteins. Usually the antigen is a foreign protein that the body recognizes as non-self. The outer coatings of bacteria and viruses contain such foreign proteins. Non-protein large molecules (with a molecular mass of over 1 000) will also be antigenic if introduced into the body. So a wide variety of living and non-living things can act as antigens, such things are said to possess antigenicity. The specific component of an antigen the immune system recognizes as foreign is termed an epitope.

Diagram 13.7 An antigen possesses specific molecules that the immune system is able to recognize as foreign; these are called epitopes.

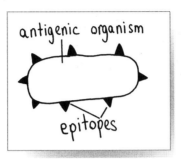

Cells involved in adaptive immunity

The important class of white cells involved in adaptive immunity is the small lymphocytes. Small lymphocytes have a large nucleus with only a small area of cytoplasm. In addition to being found in the blood, there are many small lymphocytes in the structures of the lymphatic system, such as the spleen, tonsils and lymph nodes.

Small lymphocytes are able to recognize antigenic material; this is essential if they are to mount an immune response. It is estimated that small lymphocytes are capable of producing 100 million different shapes of surface receptors in order to recognize 100 million different forms of antigen. This diversity seems to allow the immune system to recognize all of the possible antigens on the surface of the planet.

Despite this amazing diversity, any individual small lymphocyte can only recognize one single form of antigen. There may just be a few individual small lymphocytes for each of the 100 million possible antigens we may come across during a lifetime. The small group of lymphocytes capable of recognizing an individual antigen all have the same form of surface receptor, generated by the same genetic instructions. For this reason, the members of this small lymphocyte group are described as clones, comprising a clonal group. The particular part of an antigen that the small lymphocyte receptor is able to recognize is the epitope.

There are basically two types of these small lymphocytes, B and T.

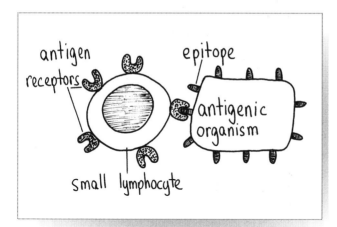

Diagram 13.8 A small lymphocyte is able to detect the presence of a particular antigen by recognizing the shape of a particular epitope. The shape of the epitope is recognized because the small lymphocyte has a reciprocal-shaped receptor in its surface.

B lymphocytes

B lymphocytes are so called because they mature in the bone marrow. Each small clonal group of B cells has one particular antigen-recognizing receptor on its surface. In the case of the B cells these receptors are surface-bound immunoglobulins (immunoglobulins and antibodies are different names for the same thing). In fact, each individual B cell has about 100 000 copies of the same immunoglobulin molecule on its surface. After contact with a specific antigen, the particular clonal group of B cells divides to produce a population. In other words, it is the presence of a particular antigen that stimulates mitosis in the clonal group that is complementary to it.

Some of the original clonal group divide to become memory B cells and others differentiate into so-called plasma cells. These plasma cells are able to produce and export from the cell large numbers of antibodies. Each of the antibodies produced will be the same as the immunoglobulin located on the cell membrane of the original B cell. This means they will be active against the antigen that was initially recognized. Antibodies are then free to circulate in the blood and tissue fluids to perform their immune functions.

T lymphocytes

The second grouping of small lymphocytes is the T cells. T lymphocytes are so called because they mature in the thymus gland. There are three types of T lymphocytes – cytotoxic, helpers and suppressors.

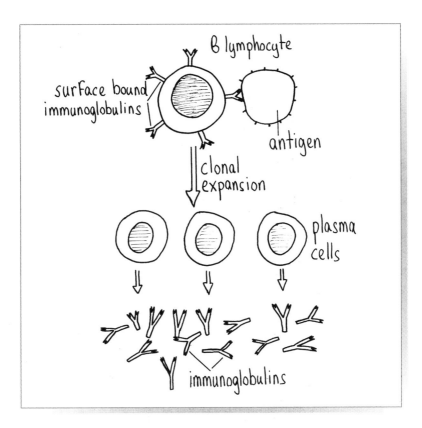

Diagram 13.9 Surface-bound immunoglobulins on a B lymphocyte detect the presence of a particular antigen. Contact with the antigen activates the B cell to divide, producing a population of plasma cells. These produce multiple copies of the original immunoglobulin molecules.

Cytotoxic T cells

Cytotoxic T cells directly attack the body's own cells when they become infected with viruses. Killing one's own cells may appear somewhat radical; however, the antibodies produced by the adaptive immune response cannot pass into individual tissue cells. If a virus-infected cell is left alone, it will produce many more viral particles that will go on to infect other cells, and the cell will be killed by the virus anyway. In this respect the cytotoxic small T lymphocytes behave in much the same way as their larger counterparts, the NK cells. A clonal group of cytotoxic T cells will only kill a body cell if it presents the specific viral epitope the T cell is able to recognize. T helper cells are also active against some malignant cells.

T helper cells

These cells produce a range of signal molecules that stimulate activity in other cells involved in immunity. These signal molecules are made up of small proteins called peptides; collectively they are referred to as cytokines. They stimulate B plasma cells to produce antibodies. Neutrophils and monocytes are stimulated to be more phagocytic. Other signal molecules stimulate mast cells to produce an inflammatory response and cytotoxic cells to kill infected body cells.

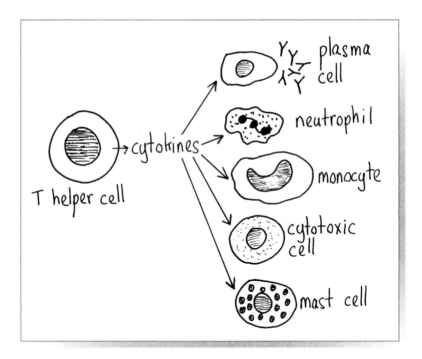

Diagram 13.10 Helper T cells stimulate the activity of other immune active cells by the release of cytokines.

HIV attacks T helper cells and will kill large numbers of them. When there are not enough T helper cells to stimulate the activity of other immunologically active cells there is a general reduction in the efficiency and physiological activity of the immune system. When this decline starts to reduce immune function, the condition is often referred to as AIDS-related complex. As immunodeficiency increases and becomes severe, full-blown AIDS results, and the sufferer will die from some infection, such as pneumonia, which they are unable to combat.

T suppressor cells

T suppressor small lymphocytes limit cytotoxic T cell activity; they also inhibit antibody production. The function of the T suppressors is therefore to limit the extent of the immune response. This function means a specific immune response can be terminated once the antigenic threat has been eliminated. Like the B cells, all of the T cells are only able to recognize and react to a single antigen. After antigenic exposure their numbers will be increased by clonal expansion.

Primary and secondary adaptive response

A primary response describes the reaction of the immune system to an infection it is encountering for the first time. Such a primary response takes 7–10 days to build up. During this time the pathogen may have the opportunity to multiply, causing the person to suffer from the infection. As the adaptive response strengthens, the newly developed specific immunity will overcome the particular pathogen and the person will recover. However, if the pathogen was able to reproduce rapidly during this period of immunological mobilization, the person may die or suffer significant tissue damage as a result of the infection.

If a person who has already mounted a primary response to an antigenic organism is then subsequently re-infected, the secondary adaptive response is much more rapid, starting within a few days. The secondary response is also much more vigorous. So when a person is infected with an organism for the second time the illness is much milder and shorter lived. Indeed, the secondary immune response may prevent the person being aware of any clinical features at all. It appears that the immune system is able to 'remember' how to mount a response to the antigen concerned; this phenomenon is referred to as immuno-logical memory. This enhanced response can be explained by the process of clonal expansion.

Clonal expansion

At birth we only have a few individual lymphocytes capable of recog-nizing an individual antigen. When a particular antigen enters the body, the few lymphocytes with the complementary receptors, will come into contact with the foreign epitopes and bind on to them. This binding triggers the lymphocytes, with their appropriate receptor for the antigen, to start dividing. This results in the lymphocytes produc-ing further copies, or clones, of themselves. Repeated mitosis in the particular clonal group means that large numbers of the clone will be produced; it is this process that is referred to as clonal expansion. The time taken for the process of clonal expansion to occur explains the delay in mounting the primary adaptive response.

Once the infection has been eliminated, the numbers of the particular clonal group involved start to decline, as there is no longer a need for a large clonal population. However, some of the lymphocytes produced in the clonal expansion process are long-lived cells. These long-lived lymphocytes are referred to as memory cells, and of course they retain the same specific receptor as the rest of the clonal group.

In addition to living for a long time, memory cells are able to reproduce by further division; this can impart immunity that may be life-long. After an initial infection, the memory cells of a particular clonal group number a few thousand, as opposed to the few members present before the process of clonal expansion. So if the person is sub-sequently exposed to the same antigen, there are already a few thou-sand memory cells from the original clonal group ready for action. These can rapidly divide to produce sufficient clonal lymphocytes to combat the infection. This second exposure to the antigen will strengthen specific immunity by further increasing the numbers of memory cells.

The end result of this process is that there are larger numbers of memory cells for antigens that have been repeatedly encountered. For antigens that have been encountered only once, there will be smaller but probably adequate numbers. For one of the 100 million antigens

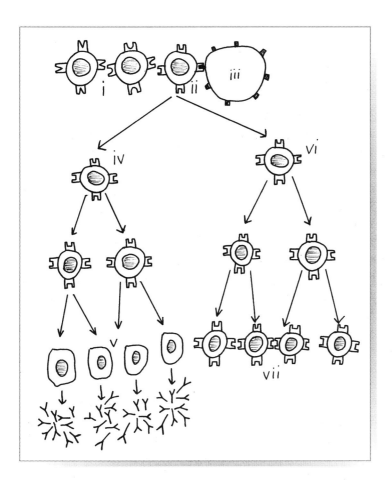

Diagram 13.11 The process of clonal expansion. This diagram illustrates expansion of B cells but the process is essentially the same for the production of an expanded clonal group of T cells.

(i)   Small lymphocytes which do not carry the specific complementary receptor do not bind with the epitope so are not activated.

(ii) Binding takes place between the lymphocyte with the complementary receptor for the epitope on the antigen.

(iii) The antigen is bound to a small lymphocyte with a complementary receptor.

(iv) One cell line of activated small lymphocytes divides into a larger clonal group.

(v)   This clonal group differentiates into plasma cells which produce antibody molecules, each one specific to the original epitope.

(vi) This cell line divides to produce a population of memory cells, all clones of the originally activated cell.

(vii) Several thousand memory lymphocytes are produced.

that have not yet been encountered, there will only be a few lymphocytes from the original inborn clonal group.

Antibodies

Antibodies (immunoglobulins) are complex immune glycoproteins; they are mostly protein but also contain a small amount of sugar. Each individual plasma cell can produce several thousand antibodies per hour. There are five different classes of antibodies that are produced to carry out specific immune functions; however, they all have the same basic Y structure.

Variable regions are different in each individual form of antibody produced by a clonal group of lymphocytes. It is this variable region that is the antigen-binding site; it is produced to precisely complement the shape of the antigen's epitopes. The remainder of the molecule is a constant region. These areas are the same in all other antibodies of the same class.

The presence of the 'hinge' region allows an antibody molecule to move its arms. This allows the molecule flexibility in binding to epitopes in different locations.

It is this combination of articulating arms and two epitope-binding sites that enables a number of antibodies to stick a group of antigenic particles together, forming them into a clump so that they can be easily phagocytosed. It has been said the 'antibodies prepare the food for the phagocytes' table'. This clumping ability can also bind together toxic antigenic molecules in solution, such as tetanus toxin. This will lead to precipitation of the toxin and subsequent phagocytosis. This activity is referred to as toxin neutralization.

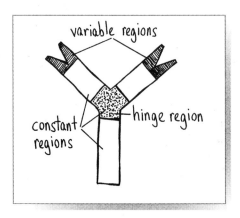

Diagram 13.12
The basic structure of an antibody.

Diagram 13.13

An antibody bound to reciprocal, complementary epitopes; because antibodies have two arms they are able to bind two antigens together.

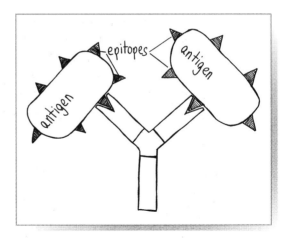

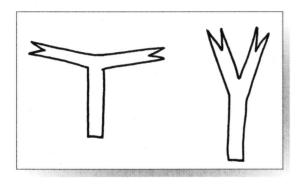

Diagram 13.14
An antibody molecule with arms open and closed.

Diagram 13.15 Several antigens have been aggregated by a group of specific antibodies.

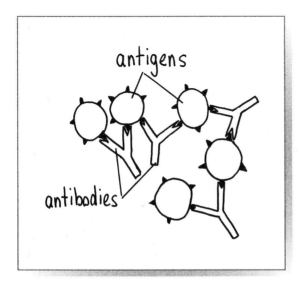

As we have already mentioned, some antibodies function as opsonins to enhance the process of phagocytosis. Other antibodies cause mast cell degranulation, which initiates the inflammatory response. Inflammation then mobilizes immune resources to a damaged or infected area, and reduces spread of infection through a tissue. Antibodies may also act as a trigger for complement activity. Some antibodies can even directly attack antigenic cell membranes causing the cell to rupture. I think of antibodies as the 'foot soldiers' of the immune system.

In the study of viral serology many tests do not look for an antigen but instead look for the antibody in the blood. For example, HIV infection is diagnosed by detection of antibodies to the virus, rather than by detecting the presence of the virus itself. An individual may be antibody positive or negative. All nurses should have their hepatitis B titre levels checked every few years to make sure they are still immune after their immunizations (titre describes the levels of antibodies in the blood).

Forms of adaptive immunity

Traditionally, acquired adaptive immunity has been described under three subheadings – active, passive and active on passive.

Active acquired

In this case the individual has acquired immunity to a specific infectious agent, usually a bacterium or virus. The body produces specific memory lymphocytes and antibodies to the antigen, which then confer immunity from future infections. This is why an individual should not usually contract the same disease twice. However, with conditions such as influenza or the common cold there are a large number of possible viruses. This means an individual may be re-infected with a different virus and suffer similar symptoms again.

Passive acquired

This is immunity the individual has acquired without making their own antibodies. Injections of human immunoglobulins will give passive immunity, e.g. gamma globulin. In natural physiology, passive immunity is acquired by a baby from the mother. This happens by the trans-placental transfer of antibodies and by the ingestion of antibodies from colostrum and milk in the first few days of life. Passive immunity is short-lived as the antibodies are progressively lost from the blood and not replaced.

Active on passive

In this circumstance the body enjoys passive immunity to a particular infectious agent, and at the same time is exposed to that same active infection. This means two things: first, the condition is not suffered from, due to passive immunity; second, the individual can make their own active antibodies against the antigen.

Clinical applications

Vaccination

A vaccination stimulates the immune system without the need for the individual to first suffer the condition. This is achieved in one of four ways. First, by giving a live but weakened (attenuated) pathogenic micro-organism which the body recognizes as foreign and so produces memory cells and antibodies to combat. Because the organism is attenuated it does not cause the disease state. Second, a dose of the infectious agent may be given which is dead; these dead organisms still act as antigens, stimulating clonal expansion and antibody production, but clearly cannot reproduce. Third, a vaccination may consist of a toxoid. These contain inactivated bacterial toxins; the body recognizes these as antigenic and clonal expansion is again stimulated. Fourth, the preparation may contain immunizing components of a broken up pathogenic micro-organism. With toxoids and dead preparations a course of three doses usually has to be given to produce a full immune response.

Allergies

A healthy immune system can recognize each antigen specifically. This ability of the immune system is called antigen-specificity. This further allows the immune system to ignore other molecules that do not pose a threat such as those from latex, shellfish or nuts. This ability not to recognize substances as antigenic is called immunological tolerance. Allergies are caused by the generation of an unnecessary and inappropriate immunological response. A substance that should be neutral and immunologically tolerated is recognized as antigenic and antibodies are produced. Allergic problems include food and drug allergies, asthma and eczema.

Auto-immunity

In this pathological condition the immune system attacks the body's own tissues. Normally, body tissues should be recognized as part of the 'self' and no immunological response initiated. This normal tolerance of the body's own tissues is referred to as self-tolerance. In auto-immunity there is a breakdown of the self/non-self recognition system. The immune system can efficiently destroy a particular tissue type it mistakenly considers to be foreign. It is now believed that diabetes mellitus type 1 occurs after the immune system has destroyed the beta cells in the pancreatic islets. Other auto-immune conditions include rheumatoid arthritis, Hashimoto's disease of the thyroid, SLE (systemic lupus erythematosus) and myasthenia gravis.

Healthy dirt

In the past few years, it has been suggested that exposure to respiratory infections in early life may reduce the probability of asthma later on. Others have suggested that exposure to bacteria in soil may help the immune system to mature and develop. Such exposure may help to increase the ability of the immune system to differentiate between potentially harmful antigens and foreign material that should be tolerated. If true, these ideas indicate that allergies and auto-immunity develop, at least in part, because children in developed countries are kept too clean. Early stimulation of the immune system may even reduce the possibility of some cancers in later life. It may even be possible that exposure to some gastrointestinal worms reduces the likelihood of diabetes mellitus.

If this thinking is supported by further research, it would mean that people in the developed countries suffer from lack of exposure to micro-organisms while people in developing countries suffer from over-exposure – ironic.

CHAPTER 14

Genetics

The principles of inheritance

Observation makes it clear that offspring resemble their parents. First, humans have baby humans, not baby giraffes or monkeys. Second, children resemble their parents more than they do other members of the same species. The reason for this is that we all inherit our genetic material from our parents, half from mother and half from father. All the information required to construct the human body is carried as a coded sequence of chemical instructions in molecules of deoxyribonucleic acid (DNA). DNA is essentially the recipe to make the proteins of the body. A sequence of a DNA molecule that carries enough information to produce a specific protein is referred to as a gene.

As genes are located in the chromosomes, DNA remains in the cell nucleus. When it is time for a gene to be expressed the information is transferred from DNA into another molecule called ribonucleic acid or RNA. RNA then travels out to the ribosomes in the cytoplasm; here amino acids are synthesized into the proteins coded for by the DNA information. Unfortunately, as well as carrying useful genetic information genes may also carry disease conditions. Although most purely genetic diseases are rare, over 4 000 separate disorders have been identified.

Chromosomes

Chromosomes are composed of genes in the form of DNA; they also contain proteins that give the chromosomes structure. All living cells contain chromosomes in their nucleus; the only exceptions are mature red blood cells. These cells contain chromosomes when they are developing in the bone marrow, but lose them about the time they enter the circulating blood.

People have 46 chromosomes, each of which is one of a pair. Twenty-two of these pairs are termed autosomes; these are the non-sex chromosomes. The final pair of chromosomes are called gametosomes; these are the sex chromosomes. Sex chromosomes are so called because they are different between the sexes. In a male, the sex chromosomes are referred to as the X and the Y. Females also have two sex chromosomes, both of which are X chromosomes. This means everyone has 44 autosomes and 2 gametosomes, 23 pairs in all. An individual receives one member of each pair of chromosomes from their mother and the other from the father. The two chromosomes in a pair are usually the same so are termed homologous chromosomes or homologues.

There are various diseases that may be caused by an abnormality in the number of chromosomes present in an individual's cells. Perhaps the best-known example is Down syndrome, where there is usually an extra chromosome, giving a total of 47. Because the extra chromosomal material is from the 21st chromosome the condition is now often referred to as trisomy 21 syndrome.

Individual chromosomes can be identified by using staining and light microscopy. Each chromosome can be identified by its characteristic size and pattern of alternating light and dark bands.

Genes and DNA

Genes contain a unit of genetic information. They carry the genetic code for a wide range of proteins. This may be part of an organelle or a substance secreted by a cell such as a hormone. As genes are carried on the chromosomes, there is usually a copy of each gene on both of the chromosomes that comprise a homologous pair. The result of this is that any one gene may be present in two different forms, one on each homologous pair. For example, the gene for eye colour may code for blue or brown eyes. These different forms of a gene are referred to as alleles. This is one of the facts that makes genetics interesting; an individual may carry one gene for blue eyes and one for brown. This means they have the genetic potential to have children with brown or blue eyes.

Genes are composed of DNA, which is the famous double helix molecule arranged in a spiral. It is like a circular staircase. A double helix formation means that the two outer strands can unwind. This allows new subunits to be added to the two open halves of the original double helix, resulting in the formation of two new complete double helix molecules. DNA is therefore a unique molecule; it is able to replicate or reproduce, making copies of itself. It is the self-replicating properties of DNA that transmit genetic information from parents to children. During meiosis one chromosome from each pair is incorporated into a gamete (a sperm or ovum.)

At fertilization, these 23 chromosomes combine to form 23 pairs in the newly formed fertilized egg cell; this is now referred to as a zygote. All of the information needed to form a new body is contained in DNA, in the 46 chromosomes of the zygote.

Dominant and recessive genes

As mentioned, two forms of a single gene may exist in an individual as different alleles. In the case of some genes, both alleles present have an effect on the individual. An example of this is blood group AB. Blood groups are genetically determined: a person with group AB has an allele which codes for group A on one homologous chromosome while the other one codes for group B. In this case both genes are expressed.

In the case of many other genes, one allele is expressed and the other is not. The allele that is expressed is apparent in the individual. This form of the gene is described as dominant. If another form of the gene is present on a chromosome, but is not expressed in the person, it is described as recessive. If a dominant gene is present, this will express itself in preference to a recessive gene. This means a recessive gene can only be expressed in the absence of a dominant gene.

When both genes for a specific characteristic are recessive it will be expressed in the person. Genes for blood groups A and B are dominant while the group O gene is recessive. Therefore, if a person has one allele for group A and one for group O they will have blood group A. The recessive O gene is masked by the dominant A. When both genes on the two homologous chromosomes code for group O the person will be group O.

Another example is eye colour. Brown eye colour is dominant to blue eye colour. This means a person with brown eyes may have two

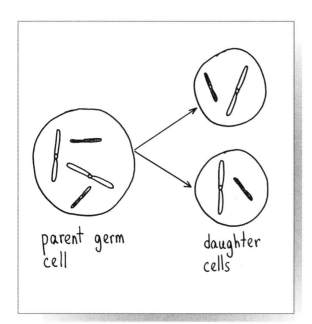

parent germ cell

daughter cells

Diagram 14.1 In the process of meiosis one chromosome from each homologous pair enters each gamete; this halves the number of chromosomes from 23 pairs to 23 (only 2 pairs of chromosomes are illustrated).

genes for brown eyes or one for brown and one for blue. A person with blue eyes must therefore have two genes for blue eyes, one on each of the homologous chromosomes.

Homozygous and heterozygous

When both alleles on each of a pair of chromosomes are the same, the individual is said to be homozygous for that trait. However, if the two equivalent genes on the homologous chromosomes are different then the person is described as heterozygous. ('Homo-' means 'the same' and 'hetero-' means 'different'.)

Genotype and phenotype

All of the information carried in the genes of an individual is described as the genotype. Phenotype describes the way these genes are expressed in a particular person. Therefore in the example below, diagram 14.2(i) illustrates a person who is genotypically homozygous for blood group A and phenotypically group A. Diagram 14.2(ii) illustrates an individual who is genotypically heterozygous for blood

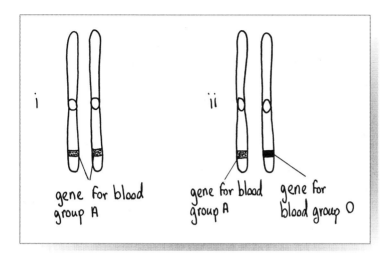

Diagram 14.2

(i) This pair of homologous chromosomes is homozygous for the trait of blood group.

(ii) This pair of homologous chromosomes is heterozygous for the trait of blood group.

group but is also phenotypically blood group A. The phenotype is therefore an expression of the combination of dominant and recessive genes in a genotype.

Monohybrid inheritance.

This form of inheritance examines the transmission of a single characteristic from parents to children. Research in this area was first carried out on pea plants by the recognized founding father of modern genetics; he was an abbot from Czechoslovakia called Gregor Mendel (1822–84). (This form of inheritance is still often referred to as Mendelian.) Gene studies in monohybrid inheritance are usually carried on the autosomes. We will illustrate this principle using two diseases; first, one carried by a dominant gene, then a recessive condition.

Autosomal dominant

Huntington's chorea (HC) is a condition that causes chronic, progressive chorea (abnormal movements) and dementia. Although the abnormal gene is present from the time of fertilization, it is not usually expressed until the person is in their thirties. Death typically occurs within about 15 years of the first symptoms. HC is caused by a dominant gene that will be expressed if present. If a parent carries one copy of the HC gene there is a 50% chance that it will be incorporated in any one gamete. Therefore an individual with an affected parent has a 50% chance of inheriting the condition.

A parent with HC will almost certainly have one gene for HC and one normal gene. As long as the other parent does not have HC they will have two recessive normal genes.

The form of diagram below may be used to estimate the probability that any potential offspring will be inherit a particular gene. The top row represents the genotypes of the parents. During meiosis the homologous chromosomes separate, so the second row represents the potential gametes that might be produced. The third row represents

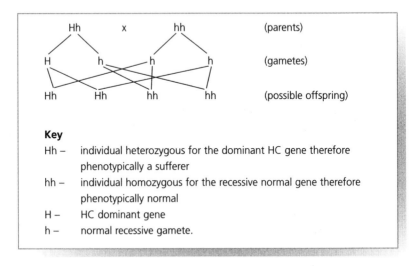

Key

Hh –   individual heterozygous for the dominant HC gene therefore phenotypically a sufferer

hh –   individual homozygous for the recessive normal gene therefore phenotypically normal

H –   HC dominant gene

h –   normal recessive gamete.

Figure 14.1 Possible offspring from a marriage between one normal parent and a parent with Huntington's chorea.

the possible children. It is conventional to use capital letters for dominant and lower case to represent recessive genes.

Autosomal recessive

Cystic fibrosis (CF) will be used to illustrate this principle. CF results in abnormally viscous secretions and affects about 1 in 2 000 live births in the UK. If one recessive gene is present it will not be expressed if a normal dominant gene is also present. A person with a normal and a CF gene will be disease-free (i.e. the heterozygous person is phenotypically normal). However, such a person may carry the defective gene on to future generations.

Cystic fibrosis will only be expressed if CF genes occupy both alleles. This is most likely to occur as the result of a marriage between two heterozygous individuals. (About one in twenty people in the general population carry the CF gene.) In this instance there will be a one in four chance that any individual born to these parents will suffer from CF. There is a further 50% chance that any offspring will carry the disease but be phenotypically normal. Finally, there is a one in four chance that a child will be phenotypically and genotypically normal.

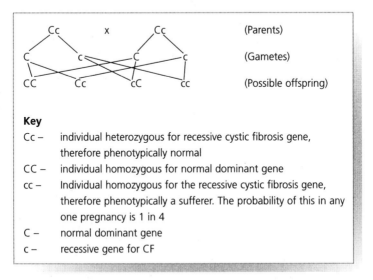

Key

Cc –   individual heterozygous for recessive cystic fibrosis gene, therefore phenotypically normal

CC –   individual homozygous for normal dominant gene

cc –   Individual homozygous for the recessive cystic fibrosis gene, therefore phenotypically a sufferer. The probability of this in any one pregnancy is 1 in 4

C –   normal dominant gene

c –   recessive gene for CF

Figure 14.2 The inheritance of cystic fibrosis. Both parents are clinically normal but may have a child who suffers from the disease because they are both heterozygous.

Determination of sex

A female has 44 autosomes and 2 X chromosomes. Males also have the same 44 autosomes with 1 X and 1 Y chromosome. During meiosis the two sex chromosomes separate. This means a female may only produce gametes that contain 22 autosomes and 1 X chromosomes. Men, however, may produce sperm, which, in addition to 22 autosomes, contains an X or a Y chromosome.

From this it can be seen that the sex of a fertilized zygote is determined by the fertilizing sperm. If the sperm carries an X chromosome the zygote will be female, if it carries a Y chromosome it will be male. As half of the sperm carry an X and half a Y chromosome there are approximately the same number of boys as girls born. In practice, baby boy births slightly outnumber baby girl births, but the reason for this is not clear.

X-linked inheritance

Genes carried on the X chromosome may be expressed differently depending on the sex of the individual. This arises because females have two X chromosomes and males only have one. Because of this difference between gene expression in males and females, this area is often referred to as sex linkage.

Haemophilia and blue–green colour blindness are the classical examples of traits carries by genes on the X chromosome. However, over 100 other gene defects have been documented on the X chromosome. As with other conditions and characteristics transmitted genetically, sex-linked traits may be dominant or recessive. If the gene for a normal characteristic is recessive, a defective dominant gene will be expressed in the individual if present.

The reason boys suffer from an X-linked trait when girls are usually only carriers is related to the nature of the X and the Y chromosomes. The X chromosome is bigger than the Y chromosome. There are parts of the Y chromosome that are equivalent to parts of the X chromosome. These regions are homologous and carry the same genes as the equivalent part of the X chromosome. Any genes on the rest of the X chromosome, where there is no analogous part on the Y, have therefore only one chance of being represented in males. If one of

Diagram 14.3
(i) Formation of ovum.
(ii) Formation of sperm.

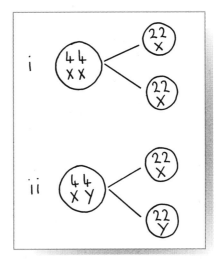

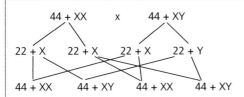

Key
44 + XX – female
44 + XY – male
22 + X and 22 + Y – gametes

This diagram may be simplified by leaving out the autosomes and just drawing the sex chromosomes as illustrated below.

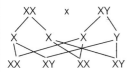

Key
XX female
XY male

Figure 14.3
Determination of sex.

these genes is defective on the male X chromosome, there is no back-up equivalent gene on the Y, so the effect of the normal gene cannot be expressed in the individual.

Genetic clotting deficiencies occur in about 1 in 4 000 live births in the UK. Haemophilia is the best-known example and is inherited as a sex-linked recessive character. In order for normal blood clotting to occur, 12 factors are required – these form the clotting cascade. A person suffering from haemophilia lacks clotting factor VIII. This means the clotting cascade is unable to pass on to factors VII to I and so the individual suffers from prolonged haemorrhage after injury. In fact, physiological blood clotting occurs all the time; for example, normal joint impacts may cause small bleeds into the synovial fluid. If the blood is unable to clot, this may lead to significant haemorrhage into joints, causing pain. Bleeding into a joint is termed haemoarthrosis.

As the defective gene for haemophilia is recessive, an individual can only be a sufferer in the absence of the normal dominant gene. Female carriers of the condition are heterozygous so are asymptomatic. All the factor VIII needed for normal clotting can be produced from the

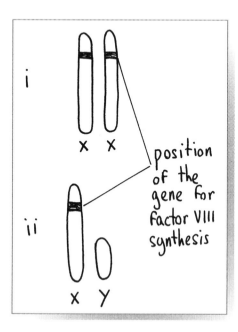

Diagram 14.4 Diagrammatic representation of the X and Y chromosome to show the X carries more genes than the Y.

(i) A normal female has two genes which may code for the production of factor VIII.

(ii) In a male there is only one gene for factor VIII production. The equivalent site on the Y chromosome does not exist.

normal gene on the other X chromosome. In other words, in a female carrier one gene is normal and one is haemophiliac. If a female carrier passes the defective gene on to her female children, the child will be normal as she will have a normal gene on the X chromosome, inherited from the father. If a male child inherits the X chromosome with the normal gene, he too will be normal. However, if a male child inherits the X chromosome with the defective gene he will suffer from haemophilia.

The result of this is that there is only a one in four probability that a heterozygous mother will have a child who suffers from haemophilia. There is a further one in four chance she will have an asymptomatic carrier daughter. In other words, half of the sons will be affected and half the daughters will be carriers. The symptomatic child will always be male and the asymptomatic carrier will always be female. As the frequency of the defective gene in the population is only about 1 in 10 000, the probability of female haemophilia sufferers is very slight, but they have been reported.

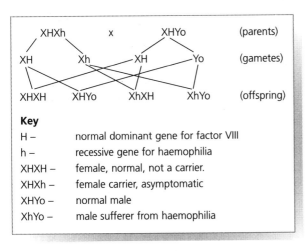

Key
H –   normal dominant gene for factor VIII
h –   recessive gene for haemophilia
XHXH –   female, normal, not a carrier.
XHXh –   female carrier, asymptomatic
XHYo –   normal male
XhYo –   male sufferer from haemophilia

Figure 14.4 Inheritance of haemophilia. Note: Yo (Y zero) indicates the absence of the equivalent locus on the Y chromosome ('locus' means the position a gene occupies on a chromosome).

Twins

There are two forms of twins. First, two ova may be released by a potential mother in a single menstrual cycle. If both of these are subsequently fertilized, two separate zygotes will be formed. These will then develop to term. Such twins may be of the same or different sex. Genetically they are no more closely related than any other siblings. Because these twins formed from two separate zygotes they are referred to as dizygotic twins.

As the result of a sperm fertilizing an ovum, a single zygote is formed. Normally, after the first mitotic divisions the daughter cells produced should stick together. However, if the early daughter cells physically separate, they will each carry on to develop into a separate embryo. These embryos will then develop into two separate babies. As these children developed from a single zygote they will always be of the same sex; in fact, they are genetically identical. Such twins are referred to as monozygotic; they are clones of each other. Very occasionally, identical triplets are born.

Diagram 14.5

(i) Dizygotic twins are formed when two sperm fertilize two ova in the same menstrual cycle.

(ii) Monozygotic twins are formed when one sperm fertilizes one ovum, and then after mitosis the two daughter cells physically separate and develop into two individuals.

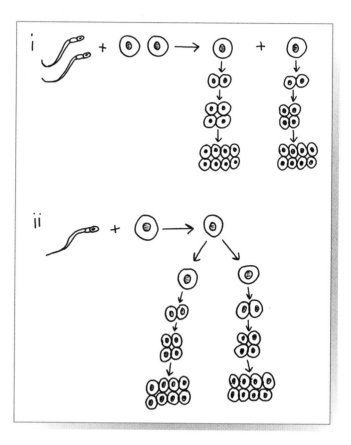

Nature or nurture

It is often difficult to determine if a characteristic is genetic, or determined by the environment an individual is exposed to. This is referred to as the nature versus nurture debate. Nature refers to the inborn genetic makeup of the individual, determined from the point of conception. Nurture is the combination of environmental conditions an individual has been exposed to, before and after birth. All thinkers in this area agree that both genetic and environmental factors affect an individual, but often disagree on the relative importance of nature or nurture on a particular characteristic.

Human height is a relatively uncontroversial example of the interaction between genetics and environment. A person may be born with the genetic potential to grow to a certain height. However, if the individual suffers repeated childhood illnesses or is malnourished, they will not attain their genetic potential. Young men in the UK today are much taller than they were 100 years ago. This is because there has been a change not in human genetics, but in human environments. However, no matter how good the environment, a person genetically programmed to be short will never become tall.

Interactions between genetic and environmental factors are also important in the cause of disease. A few diseases have an aetiology ('aetiology' means 'cause') that is entirely genetic, but most are caused by an interaction of factors. Coronary heart disease seems to be partly genetic; however, risk may be modified by lifestyle. Interaction of genetics and environment is also important in conditions such as many malignant diseases, type 2 diabetes mellitus, obesity and probably schizophrenia. People still argue about the relative influences of nature or nurture on intelligence. Homosexuality is another common topic in this form of debate.

Genetic or congenital

Some people get confused between the terms genetic and congenital. A genetic disorder is inherited via the genes. Congenital simply means present at birth. Congenital disorders may be genetic, or occur as a result of developmental abnormalities. Any factor that may cause abnormal fetal development is referred to as teratogenic; thalidomide was a tragic example of this. However, more common substances may also be detrimental as illustrated by fetal alcohol syndrome.

New developments in genetics

Genetics is a rapidly expanding area of knowledge and has the potential to affect health care practice significantly.

Detection of carriers

A carrier has a particular gene that may be transmitted to future generations. In the past it was only possible to infer which genes a person possessed from the phenotype of an individual or their offspring. It is now possible to detect the presence of a number of genes that are not expressed. This is particularly important when studying abnormal genes in people without any clinical features. If the presence of abnormal genes can be identified, the likelihood that a particular baby will be affected can be quantified.

Carrier status may be identified in some conditions by clinical examination, physiological studies, microscopy or radiography. Other conditions may be detected by analysis of gene products by biochemists. Finally, DNA analysis allows for the direct detection of many individual genes. It is now possible to test for carrier status in most of the common genetic diseases.

Gene therapy

This involves replacing a defective gene with a normal one. An individual who has a genetic condition would have the defective gene replaced by a healthy one. In theory, this would mean the individual was physiologically normal from the time the gene that he or she received was expressed. This technique is referred to as somatic gene therapy as the gene transfer would only affect the body of the individual recipient. Although there would be a change in the genetics of the individual, this would not be passed on to future generations. Somatic gene transfer may be possible in the medium term. Research is currently being carried out into treating cystic fibrosis in this way.

There is a second approach to gene therapy called germ line therapy. This would involve correcting a genetic disorder so the alteration would be passed on to any children. This is controversial, as it would be altering the genetic basis of humanity. Because of the complexity of the interaction between genetics and the individual, it is possible this technique could generate totally unforeseen serious problems.

Stem cells

More than 200 different forms of cell combine to make up the human body. Specialist tissues are composed of specialized populations of cells. Generalized cells differentiate into specialized cells via the process of differentiation. A generalized cell that has the potential to differentiate is termed a stem cell. Most differentiation takes place in the first 12 weeks after conception.

Stem cells are classified according to their potential to differentiate. Unipotent stem cells are capable of developing into a single specialized cell type. Pluripotent stem cells may develop into a few different but related cell types. Finally, multipotent (sometimes called totipotent) stem cells are capable of differentiating into any other cell type found in the body.

It is the presence of some forms of stem cells that allows certain tissues to regenerate throughout life. When a stem cell divides it produces two daughter cells: one is another stem cell and the second will develop into the cell type required. Epidermis and liver are examples of tissues that continue to have powers of regeneration. Other cell types, such as neurones and muscle cells, have limited or no ability to regenerate after injury or disease.

In the future it may be possible to inject a damaged organ with stem cells which would then differentiate in situ to regenerate a damaged organ or tissue. The problem, of course, is where to obtain the stem cells required. Until recently it was believed that early embryos were the only available source of multipotent stem cells. Embryos are, after all, people at an early stage of development. I would certainly be unhappy about clinicians using bits of me to repair someone else, unless I had died of natural causes or trauma first, of course.

Ideally, in the medium future it may be possible to harvest stem cells from an adult individual and persuade them to differentiate into the type of cells required. Recently, some researchers have claimed to have found multipotent stem cells in adult bone marrow. If this is true, it could become possible to cure paralysis caused by spinal cord lesions, heart muscle damaged by a myocardial infarct, dementia, renal failure, diabetes, liver failure and many more diseases.

Cloning

Clones are two individual organisms with the same genetic makeup. Monozygotic twins are natural examples of clones. Cloning, as a new development in genetics, broke into popular consciousness with Dolly the sheep. An ovum was harvested from an adult female sheep and the nucleus removed using micro-manipulative techniques. Another nucleus from an adult sheep cell was then implanted into the vacant ovum cell. This new 'combination' cell was stimulated to divide. This can be done by a passing a low voltage electrical current through the cell or by treating it chemically. Mitosis then started to produce a new embryo, which was then implanted to a sheep uterus where Dolly went to term and was born.

Dolly was therefore a second organism with the same genetic makeup as the adult she was cloned from.

At the time it was suggested that the same technique could be used to clone a human. However, subsequent cloning experiments have produced baby animals with severe deformities. Even if it were desirable, for whatever reason, to clone a human being this would be far too dangerous to contemplate using current techniques. In addition it seems that Dolly has the biological age of the original cell she was cloned from; if this turns out to be the case it would mean that clones are born old.

The human genome project

A genome is the totality of DNA an organism or species possesses. All of the cells in the body, except mature red blood cells, contain a complete copy of the genome. Genes are composed of DNA arranged as sequences of chemical bases that encode instructions for the synthesis of proteins. These bases are called adenine, thymine, cytosine and guanine. It is the order in which these bases are arranged that determine the nature of the gene, and therefore the product coded for. The bases are analogous to letters that spell out the instructions required to generate a person. The human genome is estimated to contain 30 000 to 40 000 genes and as many as 3 billion (3 thousand million) bases arranged in pairs. It is the purpose of the HGP to catalogue the sequence of all of these bases and identify all human genes.

A draft of the entire human genome was announced in June 2000 and is available on the internet. The final, definitive version should be completed in 2003. This will identify all the DNA in the genome but will not tell us what the genes do, nor how they function and interact. In other words the book is written but has yet to be interpreted into practical helpful applications.

The relatively small number of genes was a surprise; it had previously been estimated that there were 100 000 active genes in the human genome. Another surprising finding was that only about 2% of human DNA actually comprises the genes. Remaining DNA is non-coding, and this may regulate where, when and in what quantity proteins are synthesized. It may also increase the structural integrity of the chromosomes.

The genome generates what is now described as the proteome. This encompasses all of the proteins contained in a cell. Genes code for proteins, proteins comprise the cells, which in turn make up the tissues, organs and body. Because of this ordering, from molecules to the whole body, some have suggested that a comprehensive understanding of the genome and proteome will provide a total understanding of the molecular basis of health and disease. However, others argue that the body is so complex that it may work as what mathematicians describe as a 'chaotic' system. This does not mean the body is in any way chaotic, but that emergent behaviours and properties are generated by the interactions of billions of molecules, the behaviour of which is not directly predictable.

Eugenics

Eugenics describes a belief that the human race can be improved by selective breeding programmes. This may be done using a positive or negative approach. In a positive eugenics programme, people with desirable characteristics would be selected for reproduction. Negative eugenics would seek to improve the quality of the race by preventing individuals with undesirable characteristics from reproducing. The scientific basis for a belief in eugenics is very weak. In addition there are several problems with eugenics. For example, who decides which characteristics are 'desirable' or 'undesirable'? Hitler seemed to like fair hair and blue eyes, but I like any kind of hair and have no preference for eye colour. The policy in western countries seems to be to allow anyone to reproduce who wants to. However, pre-natal screening for conditions such as cystic fibrosis and Down's syndrome often results in abortion. This is, in essence, a negative eugenics programme – which no one is willing to admit exists.

Summary of genetic terms

alleles two forms of the same gene

autosome a non-sex chromosome, i.e. one of the 44

clone two organisms with the same genotype

dominant gene a gene which will be expressed irrespective of the presence of a recessive gene

DNA deoxyribonucleic acid, the double helix molecule that carries the genetic code

factor VIII an essential blood clotting factor, deficient in haemophilia

gamete a sperm or egg cell, always haploid

gametosome a sex chromosome, i.e. X or Y

gene the coded genetic instructions for production of a protein

genotype the genes present in the cells of an individual

germ line cell a cell which gives rise to gametes for the production of the next generation

haploid a cell containing 23 chromosomes, half the number of a somatic cell

heterozygous when the two alleles represent different genes on a pair of homologous chromosomes

homologous chromosomes members of a pair

homologous the same, as in the two members of a pair of homologous chromosomes

homozygous when the two alleles on each homologous chromosome are represented by identical genes

locus the position on a chromosome where a particular gene is located

meiosis reduction cell division, used in the formation of gametes, chromosomal number halved

mitosis body cell (somatic) division, chromosomal number maintained

ovum a female gamete, contains 23 chromosomes

phenotype the expression of the genotype as seen in the presentation of an individual

recessive gene a gene which will only be expressed in the homozygous state (in the absence of a dominant gene)

somatic cell a normal body cell containing 46 chromosomes

sperm a male gamete, contains 23 chromosomes

stem cell a generalized cell which is able to differentiate into different cell types

zygote the fertilized egg, a diploid cell which mitotically divides to generate the body

Final thoughts

My congratulations if you have managed to work your way through the whole book. My hope and intention was that the book would be read as a whole, rather than dipped into as would be the case with larger texts. I hope you have coloured in a lot of the diagrams?

As I was writing this book I had to constantly refrain myself from using the word 'amazing'. As I thought about the concepts, the beauty and intricacy of the body often hit me again in a fresh way. The vascular complexity of the liver is amazing! The overlapping triple fractal pattern of the lungs is amazing! How does the mesentery expand from 15 cm up to 6 metres over the distance of 20 cm?

Despite the complexity it seems to me that systems are as simple as they could be in order to perform the functions required; there does not seem to be any unnecessary complexity.

Of course we should learn all of the science, anatomy and physiology we can, but as humans always leave space for wonder and admiration.

Three thousand years ago a man called David addressed his Creator with the following words:

> I praise you because I am fearfully and wonderfully made;
> your works are wonderful,
> I know that full well.

Index